OP-ED
ON
CANCER

*(An oncology nurse offers guidance when life
changes because of cancer, and how to recover,
renew and to continue to move forward.)*

ANN WAX, R.N.

BALBOA
PRESS
A DIVISION OF HAY HOUSE

Balboa Press books may be ordered through booksellers or by contacting:

Balboa Press
A Division of Hay House
1663 Liberty Drive
Bloomington, IN 47403
www.balboapress.com
1 (877) 407-4847

Because of the dynamic nature of the Internet, any web addresses or links contained in this book may have changed since publication and may no longer be valid. The views expressed in this work are solely those of the author and do not necessarily reflect the views of the publisher, and the publisher hereby disclaims any responsibility for them.

The names and identifying details have been changed for the purpose to protect the confidentially of my co-workers and my patients. Furthermore, the following material is not intended as a substitute for the advice of a physician or a healthcare professional. Always consult a physician before embarking on whatever therapy or program you may feel is beneficial to you.

The reader should be aware that healthcare starts with personal responsibility. And decisions that are made regarding medical modalities are done as a personal choice. This book is for educational purpose only and the reader is responsible if he/she chooses to do anything based on what they read

Printed in the United States of America.

ISBN: 978-1-4525-9192-6 (sc)
ISBN: 978-1-4525-9193-3 (hc)
ISBN: 978-1-4525-9194-0 (e)

Library of Congress Control Number: 2014902272

Balboa Press rev. date: 2/13/2014

DEDICATED

With gratitude and affection to my patients who taught me the meaning of finding "bliss" and "gratitude" within the disease process of cancer.

To Lois and Carol for sharing that special bond of being my sisters.

To my loving husband Mark, who gave me his heart the first time we met.

Acknowledgements

To my friends and family for encouraging me to write this book, and for their help with endless hours of proofreading and listening to my ideas. To all of them I say thank you.

A special thank you to Adam who described me as being an "Op-Ed" page.

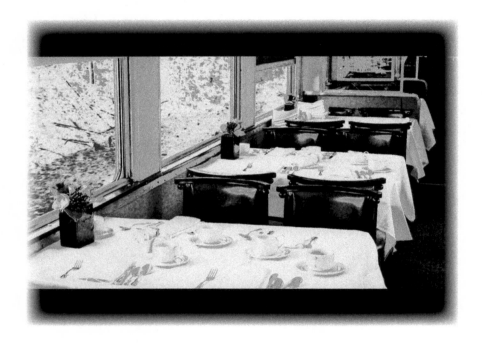

"Life moves ever forward, just like a train. Sometimes we think we have everything set in place. Then life throws us a curve and in an instant plans are changed. But just like a train that can get back on track, we have the power within ourselves to recover, renew, and continue to move forward." MDH

CONTENTS

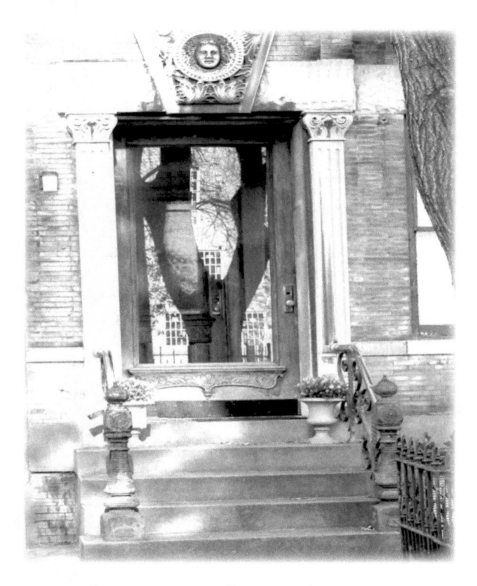

"Every entrance way offers you a new beginning."

PREFACE

How do you define "bliss"? Most people think of "bliss as a rapturous feeling associated with love, sex, or even great food. But bliss has another, deeper meaning.

The late Joseph Campbell, noted philosopher and student of religion, described bliss as a form of tranquility or calmness, a sense of being at peace with one's self and the universe.

As an oncology nurse with over 35 years of experience in helping cancer patients, I have seen --- all too often --- how this disease and the fear that it evokes can rob a patient of the will to live. To be sure, cancer is serious and needs to be taken seriously. Patients should be guided by their health care professionals, be diligent about treatments regimens, and keep their physicians informed about how they are feeling and how they are responding to treatment. But a diagnosis of cancer does not mean that life is over and that the remainder of one's days---whether long or short --should be not be lived to the fullest. To the contrary, a patient should view cancer as another chapter on the road of life ---an unwanted chapter perhaps, but not one that should prevent the patient from living, from loving and from receiving love in return.

The first step is to achieve a state of bliss, a state of acceptance and calmness. You have the disease but it does not have you. You've had disappointments in life, including this diagnosis, but you've never let disappointments stop you before. Why now? There's so much more that life can offer, and will offer, if you embrace it. Put the disappointment and fear to one side; accept that the disease is present and that you're going to deal with it. Don't focus on "why" (as in "why me?"); focus instead on "what" (as in "OK, I have the cancer.") Now what do I want to do with the rest of my life? Are there things I always wanted to do? Friendships I wish I could revive? Love I'd like to find?

This is my theory of finding bliss during and after cancer. It sounds simple, almost childish, but it can and does work. I've seen hundreds of patients do miraculous things (including, in many cases, helping themselves to heal) after they accept the fact that they have cancer, make peace with themselves and the universe, and focus not on the "why" but on the "what". This book is a tribute to them, their courage, and their success.

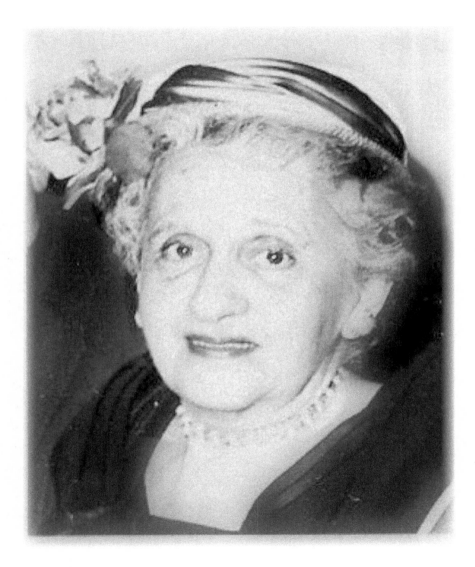

"If there is bitterness in the heart, sugar in the mouth won't make life sweeter." Yiddish proverb (My grandmother Alice)

INTRODUCTION

The first person that I was aware of who had cancer was my grandmother. She never mentioned the word cancer to me, however, when I would sleep over at her house and see her get undress into her night gown, I would catch glimpses of the two scars across her chest.

My grandmother always looked beautiful. She always made sure to wear her special bra and girdle with the special clips for her stockings. She would put her earrings and her red lipstick on and go out. No one would suspect that her first breast cancer experience was in her early fifties, or that her second breast cancer experience would occur twenty years later.

As I got older, I took my grandmother to the special lingerie shops that sold special bras. Very rarely did she ever discuss her cancer experience with me. We spoke about her long auburn braids that she had as a child, and of how my grandfather fell in love with her and would wait for outside her apartment house.

Despite her cancer experiences, my grandmother led a full and active life. She was exceptional person—and lived to be ninety. She was able to celebrate joyous occasions, with her children, grandchildren and great grandchildren.

In her own unique way my grandmother showed me how to move forward despite adversity; there is another life you can have without being totally consumed by a diagnosis of cancer.

The purpose of this book is to provide straightforward, practical help for people who have to cope with the difficult disease process of cancer. I hope that this book will enable readers to find some form of solace, as well as humor to get through their experiences of cancer.

For me, unknowingly, the process of seeing, beautiful, courageous and strong people coping with cancer started before I was born. The stage was already set for me to become an active participant in the process of helping people who experience cancer.

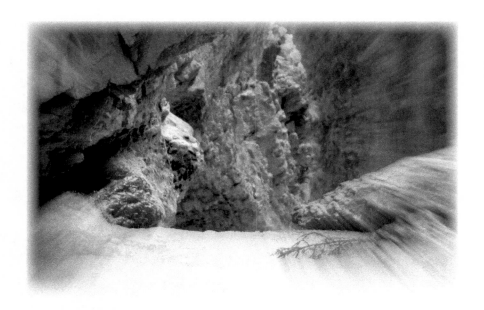

"The only true experiences that we have are the
ones that we are living at the present time"

"While man is growing, life is in decrease;
and cradles rock us nearer to the tomb. Our
birth is nothing but our death **begun."**
Edward Young, English poet

CHAPTER 1

THE RENEWAL PROCESS

From the moment we are born, we approach our death every day. There have been myths, legends and stories of people bargaining for eternal life, but we know that it does not exist. Our inner psyche keeps reminding us that every day may be our last day here on earth.

So, how does one cope with this message that we all know that we cannot do anything about? As human beings we have an innate coping mechanisms that keep us balanced—-be it denial, religious belief, humor or an optimistic point of view of life---nevertheless, the fact remains we are all going to die.

We all have questions regarding our death. Such as:

* How will I die?
* When will I die?
* Where will I die?
* Will it be painful?
* Who will mourn for me?
* Who will I leave?
* What will people think of me when I pass?
* What will happen to my possessions that I cherish?

As we have learned from archeological sites of ancient civilizations, you do not take your worldly possessions with you. The final gasp of air is the only thing that you are able to take to your death and keep.

Knowing that there is no immortality can cause distress for some people. However, for others, understanding the process of dying and the reality of death can give a new meaning to their lives. At our demise, we do experience some form of immorality by how we will be remembered. We should therefore, ask ourselves exactly that---how would we liked to be remembered?

It may be difficult to accept, but cancer and other serious illness can be a renewing process. The life that you once knew has been changed forever. The familiarity of the wall of comfort and protection that you have gotten support from has been destroyed. The process of your disease has made you more aware of what your future may entail. At this moment, you can begin to rebuild your walls. As long as you breathe, you still have choices to make on how you want to live or die.

Here are some building blocks that you will need:

* Your inner being, your thoughts and your memories.
* The realization that you have to take care of yourself first.
* An appreciation of yourself, friends and family.
* The understanding that you have the right to say "No".
* The permission to pay no heed to the etiquette that you were taught as a child.
* The concept of taking one day at a time.
* The awareness that you can be your own advocate.
* Doing acts of kindness
* Patience and inner tranquility
* Gratitude

Now is the time to start mentally knocking down the blocks from your wall of protection (or comfort zone.) You do have a second chance to change the composition of these blocks. Because of your disease process, a new insight of what really is important to you will evolve. A stronger and ever changing you will build a new wall that will have a greater meaning for you.

Over the years I have come to recognize the importance of ensuring my patients of having a full understanding of what they may encounter during their treatments with chemotherapy, surgery and radiation. All patients need information and knowledge of the different side effects that may occur as a result of their specific treatments. Furthermore, an open dialogue must be maintained between healthcare professionals and patients.

When I teach patients an their friends and families about chemotherapy and the possible side effects that they may encounter, I use analogy of the famous "Steeple Chase Amusement Park" in Brooklyn, New York. As a child I remember this scary attraction, which consisted of a long dark tunnel that would keep spinning around. You would fall and keep getting up until got the proverbial light at the end of the tunnel. It was very strange experience; you may have gotten bruised, but when you reached the end of the tunnel you felt a sense of accomplishment.

Getting through your cancer experience is much like the "Steeple Chase Amusement Park" attraction—at the end of that unusual and uncomfortable experience you do have a sense of fulfillment. Along the way, you meet extraordinary people and you become an educator, ready to help someone else that will be going through the same experience.

Annie's suggestive tips:

* Trust your intuition or your inner feelings.
* Prepare questions that you want to ask before your first visit with your physician.
* Ask questions. Do not feel intimidated by the process that you are going through.
* Always take someone with you when visiting your physicians. Most importantly on your first appointment.
* Do not be afraid to seek second opinions. Do not be afraid that you are insulting your physician by doing so.
* Take notes during your conversation with your physician or other healthcare professionals who are giving you information regarding your care.
* If possible record what the physician is saying to you.
* Feel your sense of empowerment despite your disease.
* Know that you are your own advocate regarding the care that you will be receiving.
* Find a quiet place, and mediate for 15 minutes with the focus on well being.

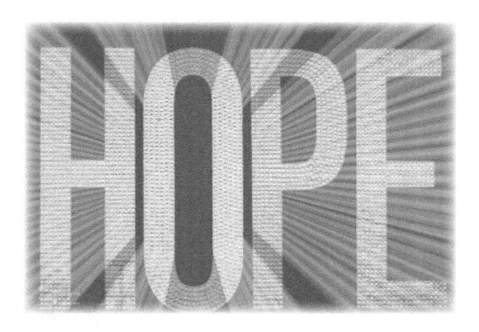

"When you hope, wills tomorrows"

CHAPTER 2

THE WALL THAT CAME CRASHING DOWN

A split second has changed your life whole life. Not only your life but perhaps your friends and families as well. Your physician just informed you that you have been diagnosed with cancer. This a surrealistic wall has just crashed into your chest. All your dreams, hopes ambitions and happiness have been buried beneath that wall. You feel that it must be an out-of-body experience. This cannot be happening to you. It must have been meant for someone else. You thought you had an understanding with yourself that cancer was not supposed to happen to you.

Does it matter which part of the body the cancer affects? Of course it does. You may experience physical pain. But for the most part it is the emotional pain and the feeling of disbelief that will stay with you. There are many questions that you are asking yourself at this time.

* Why me?
* How could this happen?
* Do I have bad Karma?
* Will I be afraid?
* How long do I have to live?
* How will my family cope with this news?
* Who should I tell?

* I'm confused; I don't feel anything, so do I really have cancer?
* What will happen to me financially?
* Will my partner accept me?
* Will I get chemotherapy, radiation or surgery?
* Will surgery be painful?
* What will be the outcome?
* What will the side effects be from the treatments?
* If I need help, who will take care of me?
* Will I be incapacitated?
* Am I going to die?
* Who will take care of, (my partner, my children, my pets, my parents) if I cannot?

Your life is in jeopardy. There are many questions that must be answered about your disease process. Fear is gnawing inside you about what decision to make regarding your cancer therapy. Your mind is like a blinking neon sign. At one moment it flashes, "Am I going to die or, Will I beat this disease?" What ever the message, you are frightened. You feel pressure of making certain choices by your friends and family. Everyone that you know gathers information for you to read and help you. But what is the best action to take?

Now, inhale a long deep breath, then exhale slowly. You may experience feelings of anxiety, anger, depression, exhaustion, fear confusion or tension. Your plan of action has to be made with a clear mind. After deciding upon the best course of therapy, do not second guess yourself. You are now moving forward with a plan of care with the knowledge and insight that this is the right decision for you.

The wall that came crashing down for me was when I received the news that my sister Lois had cancer. She was a picture of good health. Every one loved her and adored her. How could this happen to her? I sat at my kitchen table and began to cry. I knew already how her life had been turned upside down and was forever changed.

She had her surgery a few days later. She always tried to make the best out of bad situations and to find humor in them. Her husband, my sister Carol and I took turns staying with her at her bedside in the hospital. We did not want her to feel that she was alone in this time of crisis. The night that I was with her, she just broke down and started to cry. She asked me "Am I going to die today?" At first I was startled by that question coming from her. She always took life so care free. I took her hand and said, "No, you are not going to die today. Not only will you live, you will become a teacher for many people that will be experiencing the same emotions that you are feeling now. You will cherish your life more now than ever before. And you will live your life to the fullest that it can possibly be."

Lois did just that.

Annie's Suggestive tips:

* Be an informed patient. Gather the knowledge you will need to help you move forward with the decision making process for your treatment and care.
* Make sure you have all your information regarding your healthcare coverage. Do not feel embarrassed by asking questions of what will be covered and what will not be.
* When you go for tests and/or treatments and are waiting in a chair or on a stretcher, bring a light blanket to keep warm. Hospital corridors and rooms are notorious for being cold.
* Ask before you arrive at your destination if you can eat while you are undergoing your tests or treatments. Make sure you take a snack or food. It is important that you eat and drink.
* Drink plenty of water to maintain good hydration. If you are hydrated well, the person who is accessing your veins may have an easier time finding them.
* Wear gloves if your hands are always cold, and keep them on until you have to take them off.
* On the days that you are undergoing your treatments wear comfortable clothes and shoes.
* If you have to wait for a long period of time, bring a book or music that will make you laugh.
* Ask where the bathrooms are located.
* Ask how many visitors you are allow to bring with you.
* Most important, if you don't like something, say it. Do not be afraid that you are going to hurt someone's feelings. Always keep in mind that the staff and healthcare professionals are there for you. Not the other way around.

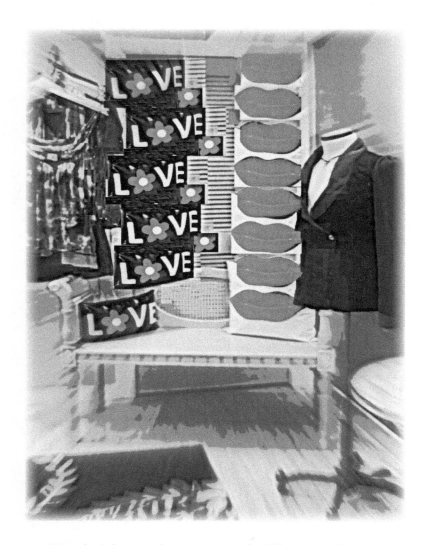

"You don't have to shop around to find "lip service" people with good intentions. They are eagerly accessible to you."

CHAPTER 3

LIP SERVICE PEOPLE

Word of your illness spreads fast. You start to receive telephone calls, e-mails and text messages from relatives, friends and people who you never knew existed. The lip service people have invaded your life. The first words out of their mouths are, "You will be okay, just have a positive attitude." What is a positive attitude? Don't they know that you already have a positive attitude. If you had a different outlook on your situation you would not be getting out of bed. Your head would be buried underneath the pillows, not wanting to face another day.

Furthermore, lip service people always volunteer information that they think will help you. They tell you about their aunt, uncle, mother, and brother or even about their pets and how they survived cancer. By telling you theses stories they think you will feel better. The fact is you feel worse. Total dread goes through your body when the telephone rings or you see a lip service person, for fear of the advice that is sure to be offered. You do not need to hear any more advice.

Unfortunately, you do not have an invisible cloak to cover yourself with when you experience people who do not understand all the ramifications of your cancer. You may come across people that will be afraid to shake your hand. Or, you may encounter people who will come close to you just to see if you are breathing okay. Some may just be in amazement that you look so great. The word "cancer" has many different connotation of how one is supposed to act, look or feel.

Almost everyone appears to have some comprehension of how you are supposed to feel. How do you know that? Because they tell you all the time that they understand and know what you are going through. It is very clear to you that they do not have any inkling of the exhaustion, fatigue, nausea, vomiting, painful tests, or endless hours of waiting, which are now part of your daily routine. There is no way that they can comprehend how you feel.

Here are some ways to best handle lip service people:

- Tell them that you don't want to talk about your disease
- Explain that at least for now your disease is a personal matter.
- Assure them that you do have a positive attitude; otherwise you would not be HERE.
- Inform them that you are well aware of the secret government conspiracy hiding the cure for cancer.
- Let them know that you would be happy to go to Mexico, the North Pole or the Dead Sea to cure your cancer. But only if you can fly first class at their expense?
- Assure them that if they want to be part of your life, they should just stop talking and listen to what you have to say.
- Make it clear that you understand they are fearful of losing you, but you are not going to die today.
- Set your own terms on how you want to talk about your disease process. don't allow them to set it for you.
- When you set your boundaries, do not feel guilty thinking that you snubbed someone's feelings. Your mindset is on wellness not feeling guilty.

If you don't' want to participate in a marathon, a walkathon or anything that is associated for finding a cure or to help raise money for cancer, that is your choice.

If lip service people cannot appreciate your thoughts and feelings, see these remarks as humorous, or if they get insulted, you know that they are not your true friends. It is better to learn who will be there for you at the beginning of your surreal experience and whom you can depend on. The irony of cancer is: if you did not have the cancer, you most likely would never have found theses unbelievable people that are now part of your life. You are truly grateful for your newfound friends, true friends, who have come into your life inadvertently as a result of cancer.

From working with patients who are about to undergo or who are undergoing chemotherapy, I've learned that there are many different scenarios that often arise. There are some patients who find it encouraging to learn about someone else that went through or had a family member go through the same experiences that they did.

Others do not.

I remember one young man who would come in with his wife. They would sit together while he was undergoing his chemotherapy. At that time he felt weak and was dealing with nausea. He had an aunt who flew in to spend time with him and to help his wife when he was receiving treatment. She proceeded to tell him the story about her son who passed away twenty-five years earlier. (Obviously, he knew already). She spoke about all the side effects he had from his chemotherapy and how poorly he did. Several times I interrupted her, almost to the point of being rude. She kept going on about her son. Finally, she left. I asked him why he did not say something to her. He said he was upset, he did not want to hurt her feelings. I pointed out to him that he needed to speak up and make people aware of his feelings and concerns about his own cancer. More importantly, by relating his feelings to people who are around him, it will give him strength to face the difficult challenges of his disease.

With my own sister, she would come home tired and exhausted after chemotherapy. There would be several phone calls to see how she was.

However, there was always one family member who would always question her course of chemotherapy. Was it the right one for her? If there was no response, this person would proceed to call my other sister up and start explaining all the clinical trials that my sister with cancer should look into. Finally this person would call me. I explained that the ultimate decision about treatment belonged to my sister with cancer. If she wanted to try different modalities she would. I also pointed out his good intentions were very upsetting for everyone. What he should have understood was that she was totally exhausted and that his questioning her choice of treatment did not help.

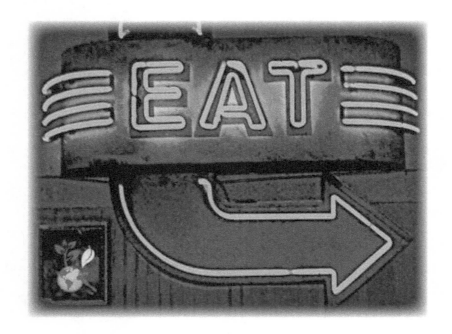

"Being cognizant of the direction of how foods help the healing process, begins with the mindset for wellness."

CHAPTER 4

COGNIZANT OF FOOD AND YOUR QUALITY OF LIFE

Food gives us energy. It repairs cell growth and is essential for our well being. At times certain foods makes us feel good. We all have our own favorite comfort foods."

However, there are times after a day of chemotherapy, radiation or recuperating from surgery when it is difficult to even look at food. With radiation you may feel lethargic and have no energy to eat. Your favorite foods do not taste the same while you are undergoing chemotherapy. And for those recuperating from surgery, just looking at food can be overwhelming.

For some, there may be weight loss because of the side effects of the treatments. At times, you can only eat a minimal amount of food; or at other times, nothing at all. All too often you try to eat, but it is very difficult. This can be troubling to your caregivers, family and friends.

Family members and friends begin to exhibit feelings of helpless because of your weight loss. In their minds, all you have to do is eat, and you will feel better. You look at your family members lovingly because you don't want to hurt their feelings, and you try to eat. Many times a family member will make that "smoothie of good intentions." Every healthy protein, vitamin or special powder is in that drink. You know that they mean well. But, don't they understand how you feel? Just looking at food or seeing their encouraging faces can make you gag even more.

Although you struggle with the task of eating and drinking fluids every day, you do understand the importance of eating and maintaining proper nutrition. Yet, people still feel the need to push food at you. Do not be afraid to tell them that the portions are too big or the food tastes bad or you have no taste for the food. Let them understand that you will find your own balance of what foods you can cannot eat. Express to them, pushing food will only make the situation worst because you will get nauseous. Your healthcare professional will monitor your weight gain or weight loss. If there is a concern, a nutritional plan will be provided.

Here are some tips to help increase your appetite and get the proper nutrition:

- Eat five or six small high-calorie, high-protein meals each day.
- Keep a variety of nutritious snacks ready available such as:
  Granola and supplement bars
  Cheese and crackers
  Almond butter and toast
  Cereal with milk
- Eggs- make hard boiled eggs or scramble
- Yogurt
- Soup
- Avoid fatty and greasy foods
- Take advantage of days when you have a good appetite to increase food intake.
- Engage in light exercise one hour before meals. This may help you feel hungry and get an appetite.
- Change the seasoning and flavoring of foods to accommodate changes in taste. Beware of foods that may cause bloating or gas, such as cabbage or broccoli.
- If foods taste metallic to you, try eating with plastic utensils.

- Eat foods served when cool or at room, temperature. They may taste better than hot foods.
- Smoothies
- Don't drink liquids with meals because they may make you feel full before you consumed adequate nutrition. However, always keep in mind that adequate hydration is essential in your care.
- Try making breakfast your main meal since your appetite might be better earlier in the day.
- Rinse your mouth after meals with ½ teaspoon salt and ½ teaspoon baking soda in one cup of water. This will help keep your mouth clean and help prevent any bad taste. (Do not swallow this solution)
- Take prescribed nausea medication. Communicate with your oncologists to find a balnece of medications that can work for you.
- Keep a diary of foods that make you feel nauseous and foods that you can tolerate.
- If you don't have an appetite, ask your physician if you can take medication to stimulate your appetite
- Sample food. Just take a small taste of food.
- Place your foods on a small plate. Seeing food on a large dinner plate may overwhelm you and you may feel anxious.
- Eat foods that you like. Make eating a pleasant experience.
- Getting adequate hydration is essential. Have a large water bottle handy. Fill it up with water. During the day try to take sips from it at your leisure.
- Understand that what is happening to your taste with foods does not mean that it will always be like this. Your tastes for food will come back.

There is more awareness of and emphasis on the importance of proper nutrition for cancer patients that ever before. Questions often arise from my patients and their families about what types of foods, vitamins, vitamins drinks, vitamin supplements and other solid and liquid supplements they need. But the most popular is, what types of vitamins should they buy or take? I always tell them they must discuss this with their oncologist. However, if you maintain a well balanced diet and proper nutrition with hydration, vitamins don't have to be your top priority. Furthermore, because of your cancer treatments your sense of smell and taste may change and your appetite may diminish at certain times. But do not get discouraged. After you are finished with your course of treatments your appetite will come back as well as your sense of smell and taste.

Seeing your family member and or friend losing weight because of lack of appetite or taste changes can bring on a feeling of despair by that particular person. My Mom and I were very well aware of maintaining a well balanced diet while undergoing chemotherapy. For me, being an oncology nurse for many years and for my Mom being a nurse and a health teacher, we knew the side effects and the pitfalls of chemotherapy. Nevertheless, while my Mom was undergoing chemotherapy she complained that foods had not tastes. Furthermore, she forced herself to eat but she could not eat. I went out and brought her different types of foods to get her to eat. I finally found one food that she liked, so, I went out and bought a dozen more of the same thing. I was delighted that she was able to eat them. Until the next round of chemotherapy when she decided that she did not like those foods. My sister made her chicken soup, the proverbial medicine that makes everything good. However, my Mom took one taste of my sister's chicken soup and refused to eat it. She kept insisting that I make her chicken soup. (And so I did.) She had a little bit of my soup, but again her tastes changed and she could not eat it. Finally we got lucky and found a food that she liked; it was chicken salad from a local delicatessen. She ate that for breakfast, lunch and dinner. We did not care what she ate as long as she was eating and was no longer losing any weight.

At some time during a course of chemotherapy, some patients may experience Neutropenia, or low white blood cell count. Neutropenia normally lasts for three to seven days. You should always consult your oncologist regarding this side effect and what you should and should not eat. One of the recommendations while you are undergoing chemotherapy is to avoid fresh fruits, vegetables, raw meat or fish during the time your blood counts are low. (However, you are able to eat fresh fruit and vegetables if they are washed very well, and peeled.) Some patients avoid fresh fruits and vegetables totally while they are undergoing treatments because of fears of low white blood cell count and infection. This happened to an elderly man who I was taking care of. He developed constipation, which was related to his chemotherapy regimen and avoidance of fruits and vegetables. It appeared that he did not understand that he could eat a well-balanced diet, including raw fruits and vegetables, except on the days that he was neutropenic; at those times, he could still eat fruits and vegetables provided they were washed and peeled, or if they were canned or frozen vegetables.

Holidays can be difficult time for cancer patients who are concerned that they may not be able to partake of traditional foods. There may be a sense of sadness that carries over into depression. Keep in mind that holidays are special for everyone, because you are there with your family and friends to celebrate.

Sometimes not being able to make the holiday preparations in your own home can be very distressing. There was a patient of mine who was very upset about Thanksgiving. I thought that she was upset because she was nauseous from her chemotherapy. It turns out that she was more upset because she was unable to entertain her family the way she wanted to. It was hard for her to let go and allow people to help her. As it turned out, it was a very joyous thanksgiving for her and her family. Everyone brought a dish and pitched in to help. Her whole family was grateful that they had the chance to be with her and to celebrate the holiday.

Gussie had a very supportive family but was unable to eat large portions of food and drinks. She tried very hard to eat, and wanted to please her family, but could not. I explained to the family members that she could eat small frequent meals. One of her daughters came with her on chemotherapy day. I saw a liquid supplement drink next to her mother's chair. It had a horrible color and smell. Apparently, her daughter placed the drink next to her mother and kept insisting that her mother drink it. I asked the daughter if she would drink that liquid supplement. She replied "no". I said to the daughter, "If you don't want to drink it, how do you expect your mother to?" Just because it is supposed to be healthy for you, it does not mean that it is good for that particular person.

I always encourage my patients to keep a journal. It is a good resource tool to understand what is going on in your body when you are undergoing chemotherapy or other cancer modalities. If you are tired or fatigue and unable to do this, have a family member or a friend try to write down how you feel or record it. A daily journal was very helpful for a particular man that was experiencing nausea, bloating and sometimes vomiting. He always felt great on the day of chemotherapy and would order a great big lunch, pastrami sandwich or a cheeseburger, French fries and a milk shake. He anticipated that he was going to be nauseous for the next few days, so he over- indulged with this type of menu. After his first and second course of chemotherapy, he still experienced the same side effects. I encouraged him to keep a journal, and to write down the foods that he was eating. He soon discovered that he had formed a pattern, and understood that the fatty foods that he was consuming, especially on the days of chemotherapy, were making him extremely nauseous. He then changed his eating habits and felt better over his next course of chemotherapy.

Bernard's occupation was in advertisement. However, he loved to cook. He found it relaxing and enjoyable to cook for his friends and family. But because of may years being on chemotherapy his sense of taste began to change. However, this did not stop him from the activity of cooking. He would bring in his taster (his wife) and allowed her to guide him with the seasoning. He still maintained his control of what ingredients that went into his recipes. He would go out to his garden and get his tomatoes and his exotic spices that he planted in his garden. There were times when he wanted the old days back of being his own taster. However, with anything in life there is always a reality clause.

He knew the reality that he was unable to do what he wanted to do. Nevertheless, he still had controlled of the ingredients in what he was cooking. Furthermore, his friends and family still thought that he was the one that added the seasoning into the foods to make them so delicious. It was just a secret between him and his wife that allow him to move forward with his life and enjoy the pleasure of cooking.

There are times when a patient has the desire to eat; however, they are in so much pain they cannot. When I first met Mr. C. He was newly diagnosed with pancreatic cancer. He was an old school gentleman and very proud. Taking pain medication and admitting out loud that he had pain was not his style. He was very aware of the importance of eating and maintaining a well balanced diet. He did this all his life. Finally, he worked with his oncologist regarding pain management. He came in the next week a new person. He was able to eat food without having continuous pain interfering with his meals. His wife was delighted that he was eating again so she made him all his favorite foods.

The fear of being nauseous and vomiting is very great for some. However, at times it does not happen. Not all patients who receive chemotherapy experience nausea and vomiting. There are great anti-nausea medications that help to relive these symptoms. Mrs. D was very fearful that she would be nauseous and unable to eat during her course of treatment. She always anticipated the side effects of loss of appetite and/or nausea before every chemotherapy cycle. However, to her astonishment she actually gained weight while undergoing her chemotherapy, because she ate so well and never experienced any side effects from chemotherapy.

Annie's suggestive tips:

Beware of orange juice and other acidic beverages if you have sores in your mouth. Dilute the orange juice with water to make it less acidic.

- If sores persist always consult with your oncologists.
- Use fortified milk in smoothies: (1 quart of milk and I cup of nonfat Instant dry milk makes a 1-quart).
- Remember that all caffeinated products are natural diuretics and are not considered adequate hydration. Monitor yourself with how much caffeinated products you are taking and your liquid intake.
- Do not focus on how much you are eating; take your time and eat small amounts of food.
- Do not push yourself to drink fluids. Try to keep a bottle or a container of water near you and sip from it throughout the day.
- Mashed potatoes are easy to eat, taste good and are easy on the stomach. Be creative with this simple dish. Add chicken soup, fortified milk, yogurt or sour cream to this dish.
- Eggs offer high nutritional value to your diet. There are many ways that you can eat them to offer variety.
- Eat cereal for snacks.
- Use instant breakfast powder in drinks, desserts, ice cream and milk.
- Stay away from bottom feeders (i.e. shrimp, clams scallops, lobsters while undergoing chemotherapy.
- Eat and drink simple foods, such as watermelons, mushroom or coconut juice.
- Drink green tea, however, remember this is also has caffeine in it. Which may keep you up.
- If you have a metallic taste in your mouth, try plastic utensils.
- If you have difficulty with loss of appetite and/poor appetite, tell your oncologist.
- Plastic utensils help to alleviate the metallic taste in your mouth.

- Plastic utensils help to alleviate the metallic taste in your mouth.
- Stay away from fast foods while you re undergoing chemotherapy or permanently. Especially greasy foods.
- Make saffron tea for variety. Take a strand of saffron and place it in hot water, or warm water. The proprieties in saffron may also boost your attitude about eating and foods.
- Other teas that also may be beneficial are: Sage tea (may calm an upset stomach and reduce stress), peppermint tea or and ginger tea
- Coconut water: helps with an upset stomach and or dehydration.
- Peppermint candies, ginger candies and or lemon drops may also help.

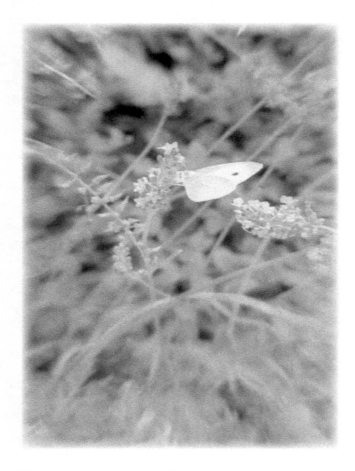

"The equation for acts of kindness is simple. One just has to be open to give and the recipient has to be open to receive. The reward for both is serenity."

CHAPTER 5

ALLOWING PEOPLE TO HELP

Your emotional and physical well being has changed because of your disease. Furthermore, you have slowly discovered that you may need help with your daily activities. You try to maintain a balance of independence, but at times it seems impossible. This can be very overwhelming and very depressing for you.

It is human nature that we want to maintain our autonomy. It is also human nature that people want to help. This is the time to let go of pride and permit people to help ease the burden of your disease. Struggling with the loss of your independence and then asking for assistance can be very upsetting. Nevertheless, it has to be done. Your health should be first concern, not your pride. Life has ironic twists: sometimes you have to let go of something in order to get it back.

Tell yourself as long as you are breathing and are able to communicate your wishes, you still are maintaining your independence. Sometimes making choices can be difficult. You get upset that you are not yourself and have to rely on someone else to do things for you that you once did. At times you even get angry at the person who is willing to help you, because you do not have the capability to perform your activities of daily living.

Always remember, by permitting a person to help you enables them to grow as a human being. Inadvertently, your disease process does help someone else. It enriches his or her life to learn how to care and nurture someone else. The one who is helping feels that they made your burden a little bit easier. When someone asks you, "May I help or what can I do for you?" Don't hesitate to answer. Give them the opportunity to assist you. You have the power to give a special gift of teaching someone what caring is all about.

Now you are into the daily routine of managing your health and dealing with cancer. You have discovered that this surreal dream has become very real for you. The various coping strategies that you have learned may help you get through the ordeal. But one of the hardest things that you have to do is to learn how to receive help from other people who sincerely offer it to you.

Mr. Mac was diagnosed with multiple myeloma. He was a retired construction worker. He lost his wife and lived alone. He maintained his household and shopped for himself and friends who were unable to do so. Being independent was his whole being. He would not allow anyone to care for him or to help him. As his disease progressed, he was unable to care for himself, but he still refused help. One day, as I was giving him chemotherapy, we began to talk about his loss of independence. He said that he always helped everyone else and enjoyed that feeling. Now he felt very uncomfortable that he was in a position of helplessness. I explained to him that receiving the gift of caring was a great reward. People wanted to show him how much they cared about and loved him. Furthermore, by refusing the help of others, he was hurting not only himself, but also those who offered the help.

Over a period of time, because of his declining health, he did allow people to help. Finally Mr. Mac. acknowledged that he was very surprised at how many people really cared about him. He said, "Who knew?"

A newly diagnosed lung cancer patient was very concerned about how she was going to cope. She was having a difficult time managing radiation, undergoing chemotherapy and maintaining a well balanced diet. Her household chores were not getting done, and her beloved dog had to be walked three times a day. She became anxious about and overwhelmed by her situation.

One day she received a telephone call from her friend. The friend said, "Do not worry anymore." She took it upon herself to set up a schedule of people who would cook, clean, shop take the patient to her doctors' appointments and walk the dog. At first, this patient did not want to accept help. She felt uncomfortable receiving help from other people. However, she realized at the end of her treatment how thankful she was to have theses people in her life.

When we experience a life threatening illness, there is an innate feeling that we want and need support from people who are close to us. The feeling of isolation and helplessness can be overwhelming. However, what happens to the person who has been estranged from his/her family and or friends for many years?

Mr. L. was coping with his cancer extremely well. He always came by himself for his chemotherapy treatments. I knew that he was married at one time and had two children. One son was living in California and his daughter was living in Florida. That was all the details he gave me about his life. One day I was making a joke about children, and how at certain times it is good to have them around. Apparently, he picked up on my joke and started to explain why he was estranged from his children. He and his wife had a bitter divorce. His children took his wife's side. Furthermore, he tried to keep an open dialogue with his children to no avail. He started to cry. It turned out that he never told his children about his disease. There are certain opportunities that you have with cancer. One of them is the opportunity to open yourself up and give the gift of communication to your family members and friends. The feelings of anger guilt, rejection, and desire for forgiveness or regret are just another dimension of the disease. Cancer gives a person a window of opportunity to reflect on what happened in the past and to move forward. In Mr. L.'s mind, he was afraid that if he called his children they would reject him and be happy that he was not well. He said that he did not want their sympathy or pity. Several months went by and Mr. L. finished the course of his treatment.

He came into the office with a young man sitting next to him. Apparently his grandson came to help him move into an assisted care facility. After much reflection about what he experienced with is cancer, he called both his children. It turned out that his children were reluctant to get in touch with him. Because of their fear of being rejected by him, they did not call. Over the years the hurt his children had experienced from the bitter divorced of their parents subsided. They were older now and understood about different kinds of relationships. They respected and admired their father and wanted him in their children's lives. Mr. L. accepted his grandson's offer of helping him move to his new home. The next time I saw Mr. L. he told me about how he attended his grandson's wedding, and he had the honor of walking down the aisle. He felt very proud that he and his grandson now had a special relationship. By Mr. L. putting aside his feeling of rejection he opened himself up to the feeling of being loved.

When children take care of their parents' needs, there is often a powerful feeling of helplessness by their parents because of role reversal. This feeling of helplessness may present itself thought anger, guilt and sadness. Often parents feel guilty that they are putting their children through the ordeal of helping them.

Mr. Theo was diagnosed with prostate cancer. His daughter, a busy physician insisted on being with her father during his check-ups and during his radiation treatments. He told her that he felt guilty about taking time away from her busy schedule. She replied to him, "who better to be there for him than her".

For others it may be a difficult time because their parents cannot perform activities of daily living for themselves. Often, a parent, out of frustration for having to rely on his or her adult child for help may have a tendency to show anger toward the child. That particular child may feel dejected because of the parent's anger towards him or her.

Mr. V. had several reoccurrences of his cancer. However, his most recent round of chemotherapy caused peripheral neuropathy his hands. He was having difficulty in getting dressed, zipping up his pants and writing. Furthermore, he was well aware that at times his pants were unzipped. However, his daughter who, was trying to be discreet, zipped up his pants for him all too often. One day, he got very angry and shouted at her when she did this. She began to cry. Her own demanding job, coupled with being a full-time care giver to her father and to her family, resulted in her being emotionally and physically exhausted. I said to the daughter, "giving of yourself is the greatest gift anyone can possibly give to another person." Whether her father appreciated it did not matter. What counted was that she is a compassionate and dutiful daughter towards her father. This demonstrates what type of person she is. Because of this, she has the respect of her family and of her community; inadvertently this is a gift from her father.

Part of being a nurse is to be intuitive with people's anxieties over the procedure or treatment they may be receiving. It was the first day of treatment for Thomas. He came in with his wife; they have been married for many years. Thomas's anxiety level was very high. He was on the Internet and "read up" on his chemotherapy. Thomas's wife appeared to be embarrassed by his anxiety level and the many questions that he asked me before we got started

I told him to sit down. I explained to him the procedures and the medications that he was going to have that day. As I was doing so, I also told his wife to sit down next to him. I told her to take his hand. She took his hand and told him that she loved him. He immediately said that he felt better.

33

During his chemotherapy, I encouraged her to sit with him and to hold his hand. This simple gesture of love reinforced to the both of them good feelings. It also helped Thomas to get through the day, with less anxiety. His wife felt better because she was part of his treatment, by simply holding his hand.

Annie's suggestive tips:

* Keep a list of telephone numbers (they maybe on your cell phone already, Cell phones can be misplaced) and e-mails addresses of people who you may call upon to help you, if needed.

* Before you start your course of treatments, speak to your physician regarding how debilitating it may be. Ask how long the treatment will be (how many cycles or years), and what activities you may or may not do.

* Do not be afraid to ask people for help. Do not be afraid to tell people that you have cancer.

* Find out about organizations that will help you cook, shop and clean for you while you are undergoing treatment.

* It is never to late to become active in a community organization (religious groups, organizations engaging in your hobbies.) Having people around you that care helps the healing process.

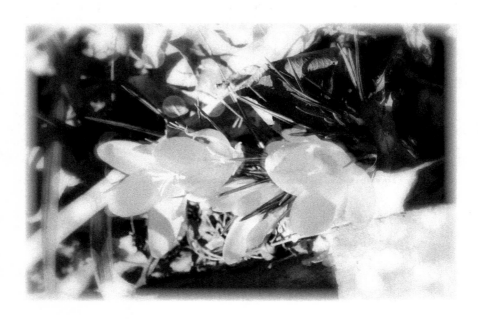

"In our moments of our despair, perchance we may
see beauty in a flower. This simplistic message shows
us that we are part of the goodness of life."

CHAPTER 6

WHERE IS THE WAR?

"Cancer is the only disease that merits its own war" (The Secret History of the War on Cancer, by Devra Davis, pg 10)

The pain, the hurt, the loss of dignity is all wrapped up in your inner psyche. Over and over again you go through in your mind that "cancer was not supposed to happen to me."

You reading lists of self-help books on ways to cope with this disease gets ever so long. Searching the Internet for the latest techniques or medications being used to combat cancer. You start to think about what types of foods you should be eating and what classes you must take to combat this disease. The personal war on cancer, you just started.

You now have joined the ranks of the "cancer warriors." Your body is in combat mode to fight this disease. A survivor you are going to be, even if it kills you. What do you experience when you are in combat mode? Your heart pounds, your blood pressure goes up. The knots you feel in your stomach. You may even experience shortness of breath and palpitations. Along with physical symptoms of combat mode, you have the mind body experience, too. Thoughts are in your mind of how you are getting ready to fight this enemy that invaded your body, which is cancer. The chemicals that will go through your veins, or burning of the radiation, or the surgeries that will cut out the enemy that is inside your precious body, whatever it takes, you will do it.

The term "cancer warrior," and hopefully soon-to-be "cancer survivor," is embedded in your vocabulary. You have become a statistic of the war on cancer. Always asking questions regarding this war, and not getting real concrete answers to your satisfaction. You learn that you can only accept the reality of this experience and go forth. Winning will be your victory over the enemy within. But how does this combat mode help you to conquer this disease? Just by thinking about the resources you have at your disposal and by recognizing the power you have to alter the course of your illness you might be marching off to whatever will help you heal. Speaking to your mind and body, as one you will fight this with all the strength you have in your body. You will do everything in your power to win this battle. Do you feel this heightened alert inside your body?

How do soldiers feel during and after combat? Do they feel calm, peaceful, and a feeling of well being? Some soldiers may experience post traumatic stress syndrome. They feel tired, frightened and have self doubt. You, the "cancer warrior" may not be facing a gun barrel or an enemy line, but you are facing an abnormal growth of cells that should not be in your body and can be deadly. This is your reality and you do acknowledge it. But how do you cope with it?

Cancer can happen to us through various means, such as heredity mutations, toxic exposures, stress, and lack of sleep or poor quality of life. It is a disease that calls from inside our bodies telling us it is time to take special care of ourselves. Your physician will make recommendations on how to deal with the physical cancer. You have to make pace with your inner self and the emotional part of your cancer.

Scientists have long known that staying calm and peaceful, places less stress on the immune system. Placing ourselves in a healing mode instead of a combat mode helps our bodies to understand the disease process and allows us to heal from within.

Working with oncology patients, there are many difficult aspects of the job a nurse must do. Over the years, I have learned that it is more difficult to access patients' veins when they are in "combat mode"--- fighting the war on cancer. In most cases, when a patient is in this mode the body gets very tense and the veins seemed to "disappear." Because of this, I tell patients to find a comfort zone, through prayer, meditation, humor or having a family member or friend hold their hand. By using theses techniques, patients tend to be more relaxed, and their veins are easier to locate.

For the past ten year, Mrs. Q. walked for the cure for breast cancer. She exercised routinely every day and made sure she ate plenty of fruits and vegetables. Occasionally, she had her glass of wine for her heart health. How could she possibly get breast cancer? But she did. However, she gathered up her courage and strength and made the decision to be a cancer warrior. She wanted those invading cells in her body to be killed by "poisonous" chemotherapy. When I first met her she was ready to start her personal war on cancer. I asked if she felt relaxed. She said "no", but she was ready to start her treatment and kill those cancer cells in her body. She knew all about the "poisons" that I would be administering to her and she was ready to take them. With that response, I asked several questions to her:

"Why would you allow anyone to give you a poisonous substance?"

"Where is the war?"

"How do you feel when you say that you are a cancer warrior?"

"How do you cope with the emotional aspect of your disease?"

I explained to her about how the chemotherapy drugs would act to stop her cancer cells from growing inside her body. Some of the side effects from the chemotherapy may be severe, but that is in rare cases. The key is to be aware of the potential side effects and speak to your physician and healthcare professionals about them. I stressed that if she did experience any of those side effects, she must never hesitate to call and report theses side effects to her physician. Furthermore, the chemotherapy that she was about to receive would enable her body to help heal her cancer.

To describe a person as a "cancer warrior" baffles me, because there are no soldiers, no volunteers or gets drafted for the war on cancer. From my own experience in treating oncology patients, I always discourage the thought process of fighting the cancer war. For me, the analogy of fighting a war inside your body to fighting an actual war has no benefits for a patient. It places your inner self in a dark place of gloom and doom.

I explain to Mrs. Q. that she needed to have a good coping mechanism to help her get through her disease process. Furthermore, it would be essential for her to find her own comfort strategies that worked for her. I suspected that she was of the Catholic faith and asked her if she had her rosary beads with her. She acted very surprised by this question, but she took them out from her pocket book. I told her to hold them and at the same time visualize a comfortable place. She closed her eyes. As I was accessing her veins to start her infusion, I noticed a sense of clam come over her that she did not have before. To me, it appeared that she was able to let go of the cancer warrior persona and take on a persona of being her own agent of healing.

Julia had breast cancer and was determined not to allow her cancer to be intrusive on her life. She followed orders very well and was a "good patient". Her and I had different perceptions about what chemotherapy is. One day I told her about my philosophy that chemotherapy is a potion that has the healing capacities that will allow the cancer to dissipate out of the body. She became very angry and told me that chemotherapy is poison and I am not sitting in the chair that she was in. She was very angry.

Julia was absolutely right that I was not sitting in her place. However, what I do know, with any negative defense mechanism while a person is undergoing modalities for cancer, it does not put you in a mindset for healing.

I say this time and again words carry meanings and listen to how you use them. By her using the word poison and speaking with a great deal of anger. Her whole body changed as she was saying the word "poison." She was in the "fight or flight mode." Inadvertently her pressure went up and her body was not in the mindset for healing. The goal with any therapy is for healing and wellness.

Sarah was an active working woman, getting ready to retire. While she was vacationing, she did not feel well. When she came home, she visited her physician who discovered she had gall bladder cancer. Her diagnosis totality mystified her. How could this be? She was still working and soon to be a grandmother. While Sarah was undergoing chemotherapy we often spoke of coping strategies. Before I started her chemotherapy she would ask her to give her a moment alone. She then would close her eyes and silently pray. One day I asked her what was in her prayer. I assumed her prayers would be for her to have the ability to "fight" her cancer. But to my surprise that was not the case. She prayed for her physician and for me. The prayer was that we would have the wisdom and guidance to do our jobs. Because of her belief in her prayers, she empowered herself to face her difficult journey.

Cancer patients who try to let go of the "fight" and find an ethereal persona may find this to be a challenge. Furthermore, the western belief in keeping the mind busy makes the concept of a natural state of calm and solitude while undergoing cancer modalities even more difficult to achieve. However, there are several ways to achieve relaxation. Some of theses techniques are diaphragmatic breathing (slow deep breaths), guided imagery, mediation and healing energy sound. It has been shown that by using these different techniques for relaxation, anxiety, fear and tension are reduced. Often when I am treating patients who are undergoing chemotherapy I explain the importance of mediation and the healing sound of "Om." I encouraged my patients to say the word "Om." Conversely by saying "Om," the tensions that they are having to dissipate and the patients feel calmer about what they are dealing with.

To maintain the body's immune system while a person is undergoing chemotherapy there are medications that a person must take. These medications often come in an injection form. Many times a patient would say to me "You would think that I would be use to getting theses "shots" by now. They still hurt when I get them."

Emily would have a look of fear every time she knew that theses injections were ordered. She knew that these injections helped her, however, she dreaded getting them. To help ease the pain, her and I would say the word "Om" together. Furthermore, there were times that the other patients thought that the sounds we were making were very strange. However, they saw when Emily was receiving theses injections, she felt better when she would say "Om." I felt as a nurse by her saying "Om", It helped her immune system by making the situation less stressful for her.

Annie's suggestive tips:

Diaphragmatic Breathing: or deep breathing from the diaphragmatic rather than the chest. (Practice this breathing pattern while you are in a relaxed and safe environment. This way, you will be more likely to use this technique when faced with a difficult situation.)

* Find a quiet place free of distractions. Lie on your bed or in a chair.
* Loosen any tight clothing.
* Rest your hands in your lap or on the arms of the chair.
* Place one hand on your upper chest and the other hand on your stomach.
* Inhale, taking a deep breathe from your abdomen as you count to three.
* As you inhale you should feel your stomach rise up.
* The hand on your chest should not move.
* After a short pause slowly exhale while counting to three. Your stomach should fall back down as you exhale.
* Continue this pattern of rhythmic breathing for five to ten minutes.

It is important to practice Diaphragmatic Breathing. The more you practice, the easier it gets. If you feel anxious about a situation, do not feel embarrassed to tell the healthcare professional that you need a few moments for relaxation.

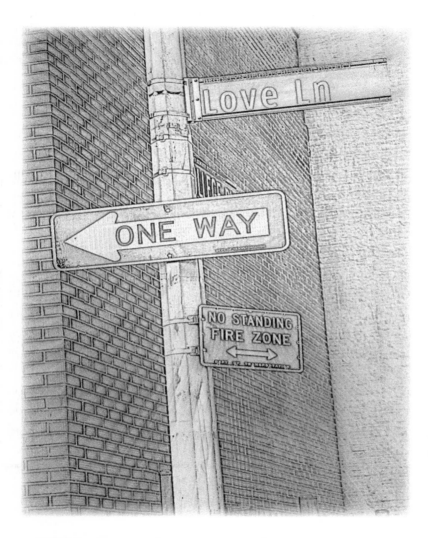

"The perception and interpretation of the meaning of words extends far beyond the original meaning. Words involved into there own characteristics that influence our emotional path."

CHAPTER 7

ETHICAL WILLS/MEMORIES

In the Buddhist tradition, there is a belief that you do not hold onto worldly processions, that everything you own can be taken away from you. However, we do posses something of great value that cannot be taken away from us – our memories, our stories of who we are and how we want the world to perceive us. Furthermore, our memories and our stories can be passed on to anyone of our choosing.

For some of us, it may be difficult to open up about our memories or personal stories. But never assume what happened to you in your life is not important. Sharing your thoughts, and feelings allows other people to be touched by your life. It is an opportunity to give yourself to someone else to enable another person to grow and learn and to benefit from your life experiences

There are many ways to keep your stories and memories alive. You can write down them and you can record them. Blogging is another way to tell people your history and your memories of how you are living. Another way simple and more private way is by creating an "Ethical will." This form of "Will" serves as a statement of your values and beliefs, background of how you want to be remembered. It can be passed down to future generation, or be given to friends to remember you by. The good news is you don't have to do this when you are about to die. Writing an Ethical Will can be done at any time. As your life evolves, your Ethical Will can keep changing. The best part is you can do this by yourself and there is no legal expense.

Here are some helpful suggestions to get you started in a notebook or journal, write down a few words or a sentence or two. Topics can include:

- My beliefs
- My opinions
- What did I do in my life to show my values
- Something that I learned from my grandparents/parents/siblings/spouse/children
- What I learned from experience
- What I am grateful for
- My hopes for the future
- Important events in my life
- My regrets (what I would have liked to do, that I never did)
- What I want to be remembered for
- My concepts of spirituality
- My favorite things such as songs, foods, places, and why
- Historical leaders and why you chose them.

After you have collected theses thoughts, write an introduction telling why you are putting theses reflections of your life together. Clearly state who is authorized to read your Ethical Will

My father-in-law was from the generation that lived through the Depression and fought in World War 11. That particular generation is noted for keeping their thoughts and feelings private. This was true about my father-in-law, who struggled with prostate cancer. It was hard for him to share his feelings about life, death and his legacy for the next generation.

Do to the progression of his disease, his physician advised him and his family about the need for hospice care. Because of my knowledge in oncology, my father-in-law wanted to speak with me about hospice. He was unsure of what it meant.

He was very grateful to see me when I visited with him. He asked me questions about hospice. One prevailing question was why was it necessary for him to be placed on hospice? I explained to him how hospice could help make him more comfortable during his final stage of his life. I was getting up and about to leave when he took my hand. I felt his apprehension in my hand. I asked him what he was afraid of? He responded, "Who will remember me?"

It was out of character for my father-in-law to write an ethical will. However, during the last months of his life, his children and grand-children were able to spend time with him, listening to stories about how he grew up on the Lower East Side of Manhattan living with his brother, sisters, parents and grand-parents. He served his country in the Army Air Corps in world War 11 and helped to build a spiritual edifice in his community. His stories brought his family closer together. Moreover, during that time he gave his family the strength to accept the inevitable.

By giving an account of his life and by his actions, he left a living Ethical Will to his family. They will always remember him.

About ten years later my mother-in-law passed away. She did not leave an ethical will either. However, what she did leave to my children were memories of how she grew up in Williamsburg, Brooklyn. Of how her father was a waiter and her mother was a seamstress during the depression. Because of her mother's talents in sewing my mother-in-law was the best-dressed girl in school. More so are the memories that my children will always have of their grandmother wearing the beautiful rose gold wedding band that their grandfather placed on her finger the day they got married, and she always wore it. She dressed impeccable, however, her outfit was not complete unless she wore her pearl necklace and earrings. Then she was ready to go out. These simple and endearing memories of her, illustrate how kind and loving she was with her family.

My mother was from the same generation as my father-in-law and my mother-in-law. She was a nurse and a health education teacher for many years. She too lived with cancer for a long period of time. As a child I knew that she collected articles, pictures and quotes, on various topics dealing with maintaining good health. After she passed, I found a treasure trove of letters in a suitcase at my mother's house. The letters were between my parents, during the time my father was serving in the Army during World War 11. Along with the letters were various clippings of humorous cartoons, jokes quotes and my mother's comments on each one. By reading theses letters and clippings I was able to go back in time and see how my parents lived during the War. Furthermore, I gained an understanding about how difficult it was for both of them to be apart from one another.

Moreover, to my surprise, I discovered that she also left a legacy to her students about the importance of maintaining good health when one of her students became a patient of mine. He and I were both very surprised by this encounter; we spoke about my mother and what he learned from her.

During my mother's illness, she and I spoke on several occasions about her concerns of being remembered. By her actions and deeds, she left a legacy to her family and to her students. For this, my mother will always be remembered.

The assumption for many, wills are done when you get "old". When you are young your thoughts are more carefree about your future. You make plans about your life accordingly. Scott, worked hard at what he was doing, but he always saw the humor in life. He was newly married and living in the "Big City", New York City.

One day he just did not feel that way he should. He went for special tests and the physician found the cause of him not feeling well. He was diagnosed with a rare form of cancer. His thoughts were, "I am to young to have cancer."

When I first met Scott, he already had his first surgery and was about to start chemotherapy. We would banter back and forth about his illness, his theories regarding healing and his thoughts about politics.

Scott always had a big smile on his face and tried to get me to laugh with his jokes. Perhaps this was his wellness mechanism for getting ready for what the day will bring. Our conversations were about the news of the day, family and his jokes.

I often would tell him that his jokes were not funny. However, he would tend to disregard my opinion about them and would tell another joke to get me to laugh.

He was too young to pass away. Furthermore, I don't know if Scott ever made an Ethical Will for his family and friends. If he did I can just imagine what he would have included in it for them. The memory of this young man with the big smile on his face despite his adversity is one I will always cherish. Therefore, my ethical will that Scott has left for me is his big smile and his funny jokes that still makes me smile and laugh notwithstanding his ordeal of his disease.

Annie's suggestive tips:

Different ways to make Ethical Wills/Memories:

* Take pictures. If you don't have a camera, buy a disposable camera.
* Use a video camera, or cell phone that can record your voice.
* Write letters or send cards to family and friends. Or you can write letters to yourself, of your thoughts and memories.
* Keep a scrapbook, or a box with all the correspondence that you want to keep.
* Clip out articles, pictures or quotes from journals, magazines and newspapers and write your comments on them.
* Go to free photo sharing web sites, or to face book, where you area able to share upload pictures and send them to friends and relatives.
* Get a digital photo frame, where you can store and display a number of different pictures that are important to you. Some digital frames allow you to record your voice.
* Buy recordable cards, where you can personalize the greetings you send.
* Allow young children in your life to ask you questions about yourself.

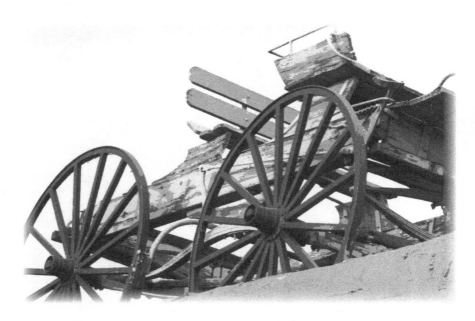

"Precarious situations may happen not initially. Still with the grace of humor, validate them and move forward with the healing process."

CHAPTER 8

HUMOR

Why put a chapter in this book about humor? There is nothing amusing about what you are going through. Nevertheless, even in a person's darkest hour, the smallness little chuckle may make a difference in how one copes with difficult situations.

What type of emotion do you experience when you listen to a joke, read a funny story or see a picture that amuses you? What you experience is your sense of humor overcoming the hardship of what you are going through. In reality there is nothing amusing about disease and the side effects that go along with it. But, even in a person's darkest moment, a chuckle or a smile does help ease your burden.

Scientists and medical professionals have documentation proof that humor is another way to help heal the emotional and physical aspects of disease. The belief is that every system in your body is connected. Every cell in your body is connected to another cell; all of the body's system, including the immune system are linked to each other.

When you have laughter, you experience a healthy way to maintain your well being. A big smile, which allows you to show your teeth, triggers a mechanism to release endorphins in your body. A hearty belly laugh releases these hormones, which enhance the immune system. At the same time, your circulatory and respiratory systems gets a healthy work-out! Even if it feels inappaorate to be laughing during hard times, don't hesitate to keep doing so. It's good for you! You feel better with humor in your life and your body knows it!

Other added benefits of humor are: alleviating feelings of anger, anxiety, pain, depression and helplessness. From my own experiences as a nurse working with patients who are coping with life threatening diseases, humor does help. Many times before I take my patients' blood pressure or access them to start an intravenous solution, I try to be humorous. Making the patients have a good belly laugh and getting a big smile on their faces before treatments helps them get through their course of treatment. Laughing helps them to relieve their anxiety about what is going to happen to them. I also found that when they are laughing during their course of treatment they feel better about themselves and what they are going through.

I also try to teach my patients that humor is part of everyday life. Even if things may not be going well for them during a particular day, there has to be at least one funny moment that occurred. I encourage them to try to find it. Sometimes, they feel that they cannot; however, when they speak with me I always manage to find the humorous part of that day. And when they do, we both have a good laugh.

Here are some helpful hints to keep humor in your life:

- Do not watch the news. Nothing has changed in the past two thousands years.
- Maintain a humor file.
- Keep a journal of funny things that happened to you.
- Watch funny movies, television shows or comedy shows.
- Read funny stories, cartoons or books.
- Stay away from face book. If you know that if you go on it and read something upsetting, than why do it.
- Stay away from people who make you upset and sad (misery does not want company, especially in your life.)

Humor helped me from a very upsetting situation. A patient who everyone was closed to became very sick. There was a great deal of sadness because people feared the inevitable. No one wanted to talk. My stories and my jokes could not lift anyone's spirits. It was a quiet day of reflection.

A curmudgeon patient came into the room. He was unaware of the sadness in the room. He did not particular care for my witty remarks about what I read in the newspapers that morning. And told me his thoughts of how I was not funny.

As I proceeded to sit down on my chair to start his intravenous, I fell on the floor. I did not find this funny, and neither did he. However, the others in the room saw me sitting on the floor with my legs out from under me. Everyone burst out laughing. I must admit it was a very funny site.

The sadness in the room was changed because of laughter.

My sister Lois had an opportunity to get away from her chemotherapy to go on vacation for several weeks. It was going to be dancing, fun in the sun and getting reacquainted with her husband. She packed her bags and off she went. However, there was one problem. She only took one wig. She was totally bald, and she did not want people to know while she was vacationing that she was undergoing chemotherapy.

That night as she was getting ready to go to dinner, she was ironing her dress. By mistake she placed her wig down next to the iron. Something started to smell as it was burning. She discovered that the iron was next to the wig and melted and burned the wig. She was able to salvage the wig. She took out scissors and cut the melted part off, she put a little more make-up on her face and went out to enjoy the evening.

When she got back and told me this story, I was horrified. But she was not going to let an incident such as a melting wig ruin her fun. She felt that this story was very funny and we both had a great laugh over it.

Annie's suggestive tips for humor: Jokes

An elderly man comes into a restaurant, sits at his usual table, and orders the usual — chicken noodle soup. The waiter sets it down in front of him, and stands back to watch him enjoy it. But the man just sits there.

"Is there something wrong?" the waiter asks.

"I can't eat this soup," the man replies.

"Is it too hot?" the waiter asks. "No." "Too cold?" "No." "Too salty?" "No."

The waiter calls for the maitre d', and for the chef, and each goes through the same routine:

"Too hot?" "Too cold?" "No, no no."

Finally the chief, at his wits end, says, "Sir, I will taste the soup myself. Where is the spoon?"

Says the elderly man: "A-ha!"

A dietitian was addressing a large audience. "The material we put into our stomachs is enough to have killed most of us sitting here, years ago." She went on to explain all the dangerous foods that decrease our longevity. However, there is one food that is the most dangerous of all and we have it or will eat it. "Can anyone tell me what food it is that causes the most grief and suffering for years after eating it?"

A 75 year old woman in the front row stood up and said "Wedding Cake."

An elderly gentleman had serous hearing problems for a number of years. He finally decided to visit his doctor and get fitted for a set of hearing aids to hear 100%.

The elderly gentleman went back in a month to his doctor, and the doctor said, "Your hearing is perfect. Your family must really be pleased that you can hear again."

The gentleman replied, "Oh, I haven't told my family yet. I just sit around and listen to the conversations. I've changed my will three times!"

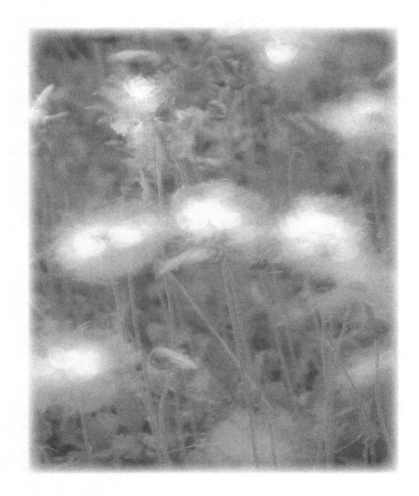

"In every phase of life changes do occur. But the ones that truly show love for us, accept us as who we are and see us as beautiful."

CHAPTER 9

SEX?

Sex is a natural biological process of life. Furthermore, sexual activity with a partner or by yourself is very important for your health and well being. Sexual intimacy makes a person feel good.

Sometimes, because of surgery, radiation or chemotherapy, it may be difficult to experience sexual intimacy. You are just too tired from your course of treatment.

At times you may experience depression and feel that you are not the same person that you once were. Certain body parts or body functions are not working as they should, or they are just not working. You may have also have disfigurement because of surgeries or radiation. You are coping with the disease process and your course of treatment, and you are very grateful that you are still living. However, it is very difficult feeling and looking at the changes in your body.

Throughout life's journey we are always moving forward. Changes occur to our bodies, to our mental state and to our relationships.

It is true, that you don't want to speak to a healthcare professional about what is going on in your bedroom. You don't want to be judged, or you don't want to be laughed at. You already had your body exposed to every tests or procedures trying to find out about your disease. Now, add another humiliating conversation that is very personal to the mix of what is happening already.

Communication is the key. Sometimes we have to put aside what will be an awkward moment for a few minutes to get the help we need. More and more healthcare professionals are addressing these issue regarding sexual matters. But they need the opening from you when to address this topic.

Some changes that may occur will affect intimacy within your relationship. It you are having difficulty with sexual intimacy, talk with your partner and healthcare professional. There are devices, medications or helpful hints that will help you to obtain sexual intimacy. The solution is communication. Allow, yourself to speak with your partner about what you want or cannot do. Time is very precious between your partner and yourself. Don't spend valuable time with a loved one in a quandary of being ashamed of your thoughts.

Keep your mind opened and be willing to explore different aspects of sexual intimacy. With a willingness to discover and open line of communication, your capacity for sexual intimacy will return. Sex may or may not be what it once was. However, if you are with the person that wants to be with you, they don't care, as long you are with them.

Ms. H. had many curve balls thrown at her during the year I met her. She was going through a difficult divorce, raising four children on her own (two children were teenagers, which added to her stress) with no financial help from her husband. Furthermore, she was newly diagnosed with breast cancer and under went a double m mastectomy with reconstructive surgery. In addition to that, she had to spend the next six months undergoing chemotherapy, where the side effects were losing her hair, nausea, vomiting, neutropenia and fatigue. The thought of having sex with anyone ever again was completely out of her mind. But Ms. H. found that special person three months into her chemotherapy. Apparently, she knew him from before she got married and he always loved her. He heard about her experience with breast cancer and was deeply concerned for her welfare. He called her and asked to see her. They went on several dates together. However, she was extremely self-conscious about being bald. She always wore a big wig in public at all times. As the months progress their relationship became serious. One night as they were kissing each other passionately, Ms. H's wig kept falling off her head. Because of her self-consciousness about being bald, she would stop kissing him to fix her wig. Finally frustrated, he said to her, "Take off the wig" She reluctantly took her wig off and discovered a warm, loving relationship with him. For him, she was beautiful with or without hair. Moreover, he was grateful to have her in his life.

Mr. and Mrs. R were high school sweethearts. She was eighteen and he was twenty when they got married. He was the only man that Mrs. R. ever slept with in her life. After forty years of marriage, they still had an active sex life, until; Mr. R. was diagnosed with bladder cancer and underwent surgery to remove his bladder. The surgeon performed and ileostomy on him (it is a procedure that entails bringing together the ureters into an isolated loop of ileum, which is brought out through the abdominal wall as an ileosotomy. It was important for both of them to maintain their sexual intimacy.

However, Mrs. R. was very uncomfortable discussing this subject matter with anyone else other than her husband. To add to her discomfort, she was afraid if they did get intimate with each other she might hurt him. Finally, Mrs. R. overcame her reluctance to discuss the topic of having sexual relations with her husband. I commended her for her courage in asking questions about sexual intimacy. Moreover, I explained to that it is essential that she and her husband keep an open dialogue with his physicians about all of the physical and emotional aspects of his disease, including sex.

Mrs. D. was living with lung cancer for two years. She was undergoing chemotherapy and often complained about fatigue that she was experiencing because of the chemotherapy. One day during her visit, she confided in me about how her fatigue was affecting her sexual intimacy with her husband. Due to her lack of strength, she was unable to have any sexual relationship with her husband. Furthermore, she felt guilty that she had cancer and was unable to perform her "wifely duties." She said that her husband never complained and only wanted her to get better. Coping with her cancer and her guilt about lack of performance as a wife was difficult for her. I explained to her that she could speak with her husband about various techniques for achieving sexual intimacy that she and her husband could enjoy together or by themselves. The next time she saw me she thanked me.

Sexual intimacy was part of Carla's life. She had many partners through the years. Her sexual encounters were wonderful and she cherished what she learned from all of them. Marriage was not in Carla's life because she did not want to be beholden to one person. She was athletic, beautiful and very proud of her breasts. Often men would comment on how beautiful they were. Her world changed when she was diagnosed with breast cancer. For nearly six months she followed the routine treatments for breast cancer, but on the inside she was hurting for the loss of her beautiful breasts. She always felt the only reason why men were attracted to her was because of her breasts.

Working with her surgeon, she was able to have reconstructive surgery. However, one of her breasts did not heal properly. She had a big physical scar and there was discussion that she may have to go in for another surgery.

With the self-doubt that she will be totally disfigured and no one would think that she was beautiful, she became depressed. Logically she knew that she should be grateful for all the good things that she had in her life. But she kept looking in the mirror only to see her disfigurement of her breasts.

She happened to go to a Christmas party; it was one of those serendipitous moments for her. She met a young man about ten years younger than her. They spoke to one another. She was extremely self-conscious about her breasts. (Keep in mind he never saw her naked.) He was unaware of her breasts being disfigured. He told her how beautiful she was.

He asked her out and she agreed to go out with him. After two dates, he wanted to know why she was holding physically back from him. He thought it was their age difference. She finally told him the reason, and showed him her breasts. She felt he was going to turn away in horror when he saw the long red scar on her breast. Instead, he kissed the scar and told her he did not care.

Carla realized to her pleasure, that if someone thinks you are beautiful, you should not argue with them. Enjoy the encounter of intimacy and change your mindset.

Annie's suggestive tips:

- Use over the counter creams for vaginal dryness. If they do now work or are uncomfortable to you ask your physician about prescription creams or lotions for vaginal dryness.
- Drink plenty of water. When you are when hydrated you feel better.
- Take short naps if you experience fatigue
- Ask your physician when it is advisable for you to have sexual intercourse.
- It is preferred to use condoms if your partner is undergoing chemotherapy. Condoms that are lubricated may be beneficial to your partner if she is experiencing vaginal dryness.
- Maintain an open dialogue with your partner about sex.
- Sometimes sexual positions are difficult to achieve because of chemotherapy, surgery and radiation. There are sexual self-help books, movies and videos that teach you various ways to obtain sexual intimacy.
- Speak to your physician if you experience erectile dysfunction. There are many medications on the market that may help.
- Men and women who have Ostomies perhaps may feel self-conscious and uncomfortable with sexual intimacy. There are many self-help books and fact sheets that offer advice to help achieve an active sexual lifestyle.
- Sexual communication and sexual touch occurs in situations regardless whether you have cancer or not. Needless to say, if you do have cancer and cannot experience sexual intimacy like you once did, do not shut out the thought process that you are unable to be sexually active. Just as the first time you may have experience your first sexual encounter, it was by trial and error. With anything it takes time, patience and practice to gain confidence and control of what you want and what to do.

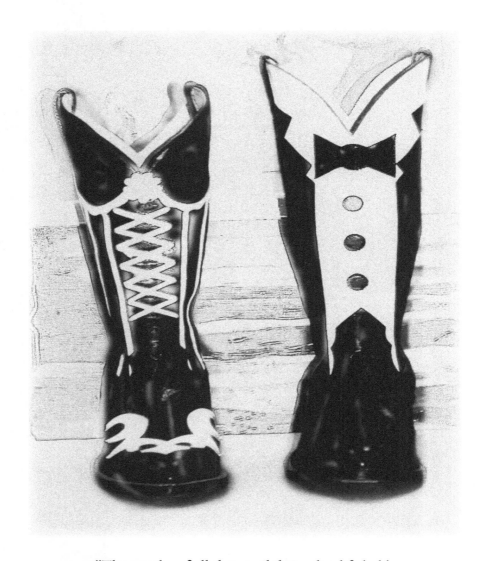

"The wonder of all the possibilities that life holds
for you are out there. You just have to put aside your
anxieties and inhibitions and take that step."

CHAPTER 10

STEPPING OUT OF YOUR COMFORT ZONE AND INTO THE UNIVERSE

Children are very astute learners. They observe the behaviors of their role models and gradually learn how to cope with challenges and burdens of life. Some of the negative baggage or life's scripts we may have picked up over the years, from our childhood, affects us throughout our life. What do children learn from adults?

- Don't talk about unpleasant things.
- Is there ever a good time to listen
- You have to be successful to be worthy of love.
- Poor self-esteem
- My parents created me, so why do I dislike my parents?
- I am a failure because (fill in the blank)
- Shame
- Guilt
- Abandonment
- Unhappiness
- Trust
- The more worldly possessions you have the better person you are.
- If you say the right words you will be loved.
- Eat and you will feel better

- Be a good person, people will like you.
- Don't be selfish.
- Blame
- Fear
- Hurt
- It is important to get approval from others.

We strive to achieve some balance of being normal and happy in our adult life. However, the negative baggage from our childhood gets heavy as we take our positions into the reality of adulthood. Every time we try to rid ourselves of the behavior that we learned as children, those negative thoughts creep up on us and we tend to feel uncomfortable.

- Am I loved?
- Am I a selfish person?
- Who do I have to please to get approval?
- Why I am I stupid?
- Why am I a failure?
- I am not good enough
- Why am I an outsider to those who love me?
- Why must I keep secrets about my family?
- Why do I bring shame on my family?

It does not matter how old you are or how successful you may be. Those feelings are there. You become that small child again and the pain is there with you. You try hard to rid of that pain, but it is persistent and it stays. Not only does it affect your whole being, but it also affects your relationship with the people around you.

When we are in a crisis situation, these feelings and thoughts surface into our conscious minds. We resort to the coping mechanisms that we learned as children.

But now, it is even more difficult to tolerate the heavy burden of what was in that baggage. All the feelings of "what if," "why me?" (but why not you?) or "What does this all mean?" escalate in our minds.

Stop these negative feelings. This is your chance to grow as a person. It is your time to fully open that baggage and to take out what you want from your life experiences and to discard the toxic lessons of the past. Pay attention to what is going on around you and what is going inside you.

Listen and feel your inner psyche. Change your life today. Don't dwell on yesterday. It is gone, and you are never going to get it back. You don't know what your future will hold. You and everyone else only have today. The only difference with a cancer patient is, that you face your mortality in a more realistic way then most others.

Today is the day that you can change your life. Don't say, "try", because when you say, "try" it already means self-doubt. You are going to take control of your life for however short or long it may be. And whatever you do, don't look back at your life with regrets. That is wasted energy, negative energy. You are moving forward to being that unique person who happens to have cancer, or the person who had cancer and is now living a cancer free fulfilling life.

There are many components that make up who we are as individuals, such as the passing of narrative stories of the hardships that our parents or grandparents endured, our genetic composition, and the high points and the low points in our lives. All of theses components weave various patterns together form the fabric of who we are. At times, we make attempts to change the destructive patterns that may form from our life experiences. Nevertheless, these destructive patterns persist through out our lives; at times they may cause great emotional harm to our inner psyche. Furthermore, for some of us, the struggle to change is an uphill battle even though we know that the outcome is for our own well being. As a nurse, I have seen patients grappling with destructive and painful patterns of behavior because of life experiences. Although it appears inconceivable, getting a diagnosis of cancer can give a person the tools to change his/her life.

Zenia was petrified about the prognosis for her disease, because she was the caretaker for her husband and her two adult children. She was afraid that her family would be unable to take care of themselves without her. Besides worrying about her family, her evenings were composed of friends calling on the telephone, to tell her about their problems. By the time she was ready to go to bed at night she was emotionally exhausted from dealing with her cancer and from everyone around her. However, she soon discovered that if she locked herself in her bathroom, no one would bother her. Hence, her bathroom became her sanctuary of peace and tranquility. One day she opened up to me about the comical situation of finding solitude in one's own bathroom. But she also expressed anger at herself, for allowing people to take advantage of her time, especially when she was tired and fatigued from her chemotherapy.

Over a period of months, I soon learned that Zenia lost her mother at an early age and was the oldest of four siblings. She was expected to cook, clean, shop take care of her younger siblings and go to school. At the age of eighteen she got a job and shortly thereafter got married. Even though she was a wife, it was assumed that she would still make financial contribution towards the well being of her father and siblings. The role of being the designated caregiver from a young age continued well into her adult years, except now she had the added burden of being a caregiver for her husband and children. Another component that was woven into her personal fabric was guilt. She felt guilty that she did not spend quality time with her husband and children, because she was always working at a job she hated. The third component was remorse, for pursing the activities she found pleasure in.

During her quiet moments in her bathroom, she slowly began to realize how her life was consumed by everyone else's needs but not her own.

Moreover, by living with her cancer she discovered that it was more important for her to take care of her needs first.

At the end of her chemotherapy, she was very grateful that she experienced cancer. Conversely, the cancer was a "wake-up call" for her to let go of the guilt and the remorse that she held inside of her since she was a child. More importantly, she found her inner strength and was no longer afraid of her prognosis.

Mr. C. was of Irish descent. He had a blue collar job, lived with his wife and six children, paid his bills and occasionally would make his appearance at church when his wife would ask him to go. In his eyes, he lived his life as a man was supposed to. No matter how difficult life's challenges were, he would get through them (as he always did in the past). Six months he retired from his job at the age of 65, he started to experience difficulty in swallowing solid foods along with a foul breath odor. His family became alarmed when they saw that he was slowly losing weight during this period of time. They pleaded with him to see a physician to check out his symptoms. He became argumentative with his family and kept insisting that there as nothing wrong with him. But after six months, he began to cough up bright red blood and drove himself to the local emergency room. After taking many tests, the doctors suspected that he had esophageal cancer. They told him that in order for them to make an accurate diagnosis, there were further tests that would have to be performed and that he must tell his family.

Mr. C. underwent surgery and adjuvant chemotherapy. While he was undergoing chemotherapy he experienced many side effects. However, he was raised to face life's challenges and not to complain because he was a man. Soon his family members became his advocates and spoke to his physician and nurses about the effects of his chemotherapy. But, Mr. C. slowly began to spiral into the black hole of depression, because of what was happening to him. The healthcare team and his family members encouraged him to seek psychotherapy, but he refused. Furthermore, this suggestion only increases his depression even more.

His wife finally contacted the local parish priest who was non-threatening towards Mr.C.. The priest would come and visit with Mr.C. two times a week in his home. At first they only spoke about baseball and the Yankees. As the days progressed, the subject matter changed to family, what type of work Mr. C. did before retirement, humor, music, his active duty in the army, and religion. Finally, the priest asked him what his fears were thinking that the answer would be about dying. Mr. C. explained to the priest that he expected to have a good outcome with his cancer and he was not afraid of dying if that should happen. Because of his family's attention and love, he felt undeserving of them.

Apparently, Mr. C. had a father who was an alcoholic and was abusive towards him as a child. When he was a teenager, he got into a brutal fight with his father and had to move out of his home. Over the years, he lost contact with his father, until he received a telephone call from his father explaining that he was dying and that he would like to see him. Due to his anger and feelings the old wounds he had suffered as a child Mr. C. never went to visit his dying father. For all theses years, he carried the emptiness inside of him of not saying goodbye to his father.

Finally, Mr. C. burden of remorse was out in the open. By speaking to his priest about this difficult time in his life with his father, it enabled Mr. C. to unlock the sorrow that he had inside with his father. Now, as an adult, he gained insight about his relationship with is father. He comprehended that the blame for lack of communication with his father was his father's personality, not his. Furthermore, he understood that his father should have acted as a parent toward him throughout his life. Moreover, it was time for him now to allow the emptiness that was inside of him to be filled with the love from his family. From that day forward, Mr. C. was able to accept his family's love with all his heart.

Al too often, I have seen cancer patients at the beginning of their diagnosis afraid to tell their healthcare team, family members, friends and people in their community of how they feel and what they need from them. I explain to the patients that cancer does not take away their ability to communicate with others. Hence, cancer teaches you "I, myself, matter." Therefore, by comprehending that thought process, you gain lessons of courage, humility, love and strength to enhance your well being

The ever-changing world for Mrs. L. challenged her inner comfort zone. Before she was born, her grandparents were sent to Siberia because of disagreements with the Communist government for helping Jews. As a child they would tell stories of what her community was like before the communist took over. Her peaceful childhood was destroyed by the untimely death of her mother. When she started school she was penalized because of her grandparents past. Quickly she learned not to question, not to give an opinion; she learned that if you do, you will be punished. Because she excelled in sports, she was able to travel to different places in the world. But that world changed, too because of the downfall of the communist party in her country. At that point in her life, she had to accept another change.

However, an opportunity arose for her and her husband to come to the United States. With very little money and minimal knowledge of the English language, she and her husband decided to make a new life in the United States. Mrs. L. was working long hours at her job. One day she felt a sharp pain in her abdomen, but she ignored it, because she was taught to hide pain. Then some days later the pain was much worse. Her husband rushed her to the hospital, where a surgical oncologist discovered that she had uterine cancer. Again, her world changed. This time her life was involved.

I met Mrs. L. after she had surgery, when she was getting ready to start chemotherapy. She was very quiet and did not ask many questions. Over the course of her chemotherapy treatments, I learned about her past history. I discovered that it was difficult for her to express her feelings, for fear that she would get into trouble if she did. I encouraged her to "open her mouth", to say what she felt. This was totally a new concept for her. Slowly over time, she gained an inner power to do just that.

Her cancer gave her the autonomy to be her own person. She had a new world of freedom. Now, she is an American citizen and an owner of a small business.

During my many years taking care of cancer patients, I often ask questions about how they grew up, are they married, how many siblings do they have, what type of job do they do, and various other questions. I always thought it was odd that other nurses, who are taking care of the same patients , knew very little about them. Furthermore, learning about their trials and tribulations of life also helped me find emotional healing tools to help them through these difficult times. Often the patients would ask me if I was a "therapist". I would reply, "No, I am not." However, I am an observer of human emotions of people going through tumultuous times in their lives. By me asking questions about them, I gained the emotional tools that I needed to help them. With theses tools that I acquired from them I was able to be a better nurse for them.

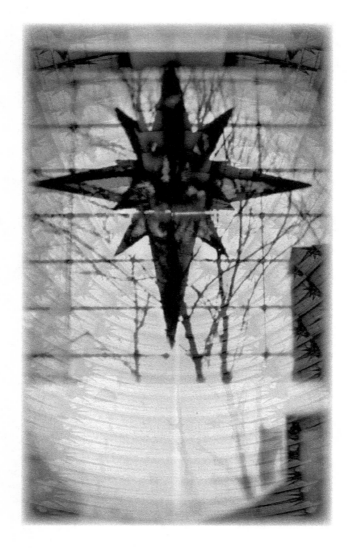

"Unkind words penetrate out intuitive self. For
our protection, we do not react to them, we just
buried them deep inside, so they won't hurt."

CHAPTER 11

WORDS

Words have intrinsic meanings for us. But how often do we take the time to listen to the words that we use and to hear words that are spoken to us by others. All too often we speak not realizing what we are saying to ourselves and to others. Furthermore, do we comprehend that every word has a meaning that may affect us both physically and emotionally in our daily lives and in our future?

Here is a simple experiment that shows how words not only affect our minds but they also affect us physically as well. Try closing your eyes and have someone describe to you the smell and taste of a lemon. Your senses will begin to work with just only those words that are being used to describe the lemon. Water will fill your mouth and you can taste the bitterness of the lemon.

Our five senses are affected by the words we speak and by the words that we see and hear. Many times we don't give a second thought to the importance of them until we stop and see the affects they have on us. Subconsciously our feelings and energy are creative in our minds because of words. We know this to be true, because of the way we feel and our reaction to things. Example, you just finished a great book with a happy ending and you feel good about the book, or you read a newspaper article about violence in the world and you become angry and upset.

Furthermore, when hateful or derogatory words are spoken to us, a universal feeling of inadequacy or shame comes over us. On the other hand, perhaps a kind remark of doing a good a job makes us feel worthy. Or someone tells you that they "love you" and you feel good. Simple conversations on a simple level of understanding of words do have a deep profound affect on our emotional and physical well-being.

The word love has its own special meanings. This affects our inner psyche. One may look for the right person to spend their life with, however, you discovered it was not so. Another type of love is the love between a parent and a child. It is binding by words and actions. But how often does the child feel the "love"?

Another word I hear often is "Please". Many conversations have the components that people must "please" someone else. I say what about pleasing yourself. Why do you have to give up what you want, so you can "please" someone else? Are you living their life? Why do you have to put aside your feelings to "please" another person?

Compromises are to be made. And there is nothing wrong in that. However, all too often the person who is making compromises is usually doing it to please another person. You are not a selfish person if you express your thoughts and wishes of what you want in your own words.

Our inner psyche carries around certain words that were reinforce to us when we were children. Of whom we are and how we are supposed to behave. Furthermore, there are times when the mindset of these words can overpower us and lead us to unhealthy behaviors that are not good for our health.

We may say phrases of words to form wishes, or expectations with hope to improve our lives. We put out words and hope that they will come true. I often say be careful what you wish for, because you may receive it. However, not in the form you expected it to come in. How often do we say, "I wish I had a million dollars?" Getting cancer and the costs of tests, treatments and care may well be over a million dollars for many. Your wish of getting that money did come to you, but not in the way you wanted it.

From my relationships with family, friends, co-workers and my patients I have realized words do take on meanings of their own. Perhaps this is because of our perception and interpretation of our own life's experiences that we incorporate in their meanings. Such as these simple words, mother, father. The meanings of these words can be endless, because of the importance of them and how they affect us emotionally.

Judith was a devoted mother, sister, wife and friend. She grew up in a culture where women were taught to have "peace" in the home. Her husband made the decisions and she had to live by them. Because of the turmoil of her native country she had to resettle in the United Sates.

Her family adored her because she was the peacemaker in the home. With the transition move to New York City, she helped her family get through a difficult time without expressing her fears and anxieties of what she was going through. She kept silent, for she did not want to upset them.

Sitting with her and listening to her story of how difficult the move was to the Untied Sates, and the stress of it, she felt that her cancer evolved from that. But was that the only reason? Even though her family was extremely supportive of her during her course of treatments. From time to time there would be a family member that would show up that would distress her.

She knew ahead of time about them coming to visit her, but would not tell them not to come. She did not want to upset them. Here she was putting aside her feelings. She had to keep peace and harmony in the family.

I told her that words do set you free. She longer had to be the peacekeeper in her family or try to please someone else. She had the cancer not them.

She was going through difficult times not them. If she did not want them to visit her, say it. I joked with Judith, I said, "Perhaps they will not get the meaning of your words, and they will visit anyway." She did tell them that she was too tired for their visit, and they did visit her anyway.

Liz was a people pleaser. She was raised in a house where you had to do what you were told in order to get love. If you wanted something put your feelings aside and do what you were told. That is how you would get the love that you wanted. Her wish was to get out of her house as soon as possible, go to college and marry the "right person" and live happily ever after.

Her wishes came true. At the age if eighteen she left home for college. Got married to the "right" person that her parents' thought was good for her. (She did love him, until she learned what he was like after she was married.) She had a child and lived in the suburbs in a beautiful home.

Life appeared to be good on the outside. She soon discovered that he was abusive verbally and physically towards her. Liz's parents encouraged her to stay in the relationship and just ignored his words and stay out of his way. He was wealthy and she appeared to live a great life.

However, her intuitive self, knew that the longer she stayed with him the sicker she was getting. She gathered the courage to take her child and move out. Her parents were upset because now they had to explain to their friends and family that the picture perfect marriage was not so perfect.

Liz got her divorced and made a life for her and her child. She managed to get a good job. To her credit she overlooked her parents viewpoints of what she did wrong in the marriage and was a dutiful daughter to them.

She always was a giving person and thinking of others. So much so, she overlooked to what was happening to her own body. Her intuitive self finally made her seek out a physician to check out why she was so fatigue.

When she got the diagnosed of colon cancer, she was not surprised. She felt that all her life she was always containing sewage in her body and had difficulty letting it go.

Because of her wonderful and giving heart she had very good friends who loved her very much. Her fear was of hurting people's feelings with her words and actions.

Finally Liz and I had a discussion one day about saying "no" to people and making yourself the first priority in your life.

I explained to her, if she was not well, than she would not be able to help her friends when they needed her. At first she was reluctance to live by this philosophy. However, the more time I spent with her and reinforcing with words of how important it was for her to take care of herself, she finally listened.

Words are so profound and I keep reinforcing this with my patients. One day Sherri came in for chemotherapy. She was disheartened by how her treatments were going. She had cancer once before and this should not have been a reoccurrence. In spite of her cancer she was in good health. She made this statement, "I just want it o be over." I told her to clarify your statement, "Don't say I want it to be over." Rephrase what you just said and think about your words that you are putting out into the universe. She paused, said that "I was right", and changed her statement. Now, her words include wellness, health, and contentment.

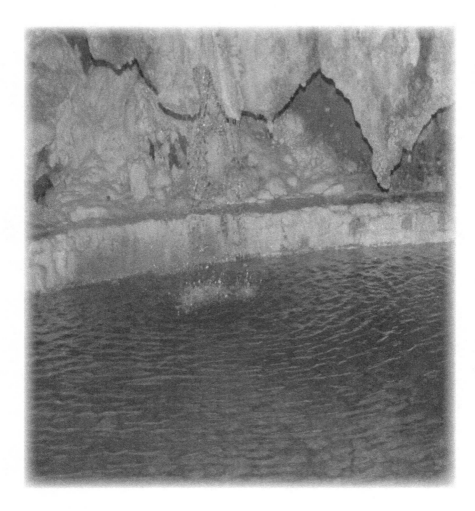

"The natural source of your spirituality involves
the past, the present and the future. The connection
of all three is the harmony of self."

CHAPTER 12

THE CLOTH OF YOUR
WELL BEING?

Listening to patients talk about their family backgrounds, how they were raised, their spiritual thoughts and even how they were disciplined, I often see a pattern of how one generation influences the next. These influences may include ancestral stories, family emotional upheaval, physical frailties, and what a person perceives is expected of him/her, regarding family and community. Each individual weaves a certain emotional cloth that is just underneath the conscious mind. Your thoughts and actions are governed by your ancestral past, even though you may not be aware of this energy that is inside you. Usually, it occurs in a silent or quiet way without being recognized by the conscious mind.

The shape, the size, and the texture gives you, the weaver, a specific cloth of your own. The emotional cloth may enhance an experience or may cause harm. Because you can't let it go. All too often, what may emerge from being the recipient of this particular cloth is an emotional and or physical disease process or malady that can cause harm to the immune system.

These patterns of thought affect every cell in our bodies and can change the immune system for healing or for sickness. Time and again, I have suggested to my patients, with humor, that we all need an "emotional sewage treatment plant in our bodies". This emotional plant can take what is needed from good thoughts that are going through our bodies and discard the ones that are hazardous to us. Often there is a small smile and a moment's pause and the patient will say, "You know, you are right. But how I am supposed to do this? It is so difficult for me." I tell them they must start at that very moment of conscious thought. The process of cleansing one's emotional cloth is essential for wellness. Nevertheless, people find it an extremely difficult task to perform.

The other expression that I often use is, "It is time to grow up." Age, maturity, wealth or status does not make you a "grown person". It may make you functional and successful, but your emotional maturity inside can still be that small child. The time when you are a "grown up" is when you acknowledged that those who made you feel guilty, angry or hurt, are no longer in control of your life or your thought process. Harboring theses negative feelings (even in your subconscious mind) affects your health and wellbeing and takes a toll on your health.

Over and over again, people ask me jokingly, "Ann, when do you know that you are a grown up?" I respond, "The moment there is no longer a feeling that you are not good enough. When no one can make you feel guilty or control you regarding what you do or do not do." Furthermore, "When you wholeheartedly feel that you are worthy of hugging yourself with the understanding that you are truly good, without the acknowledgement from someone else."

I often tell people that they should give themselves a hug everyday. When you wake up from your sleep, acknowledged that you are a good, kind, and loving and important person in this universe. Furthermore, do not forget a big kiss as well to yourself for being you. For if you don't think that you are worthy of this admiration of self how can you accept it from others?

Jocelyn was born into a chaotic, dysfunctional family. She had many sisters and one brother. She was known as the diplomat of the family.

She made sure everyone got along with each other. Furthermore, when someone was sick or needed help, at a moment's notice she was there to help. Jocelyn placed her needs on the back burner, hoping that one day she could attend to them.

Her parents taught her to cope with adversity, to keep her emotions deep inside of herself, and nurture others despite how they may have hurt her. These were the threads that were woven into her life's cloth. Maintaining an unhealthy lifestyle of smoking and staying in abusive relationships were her additional components to the cloth. She confided in me, that this behavior she felt lowered her resistance to illness.

Jocelyn had a tempestuous relationship with her brother. She had panic attacks, severe anxiety, and reoccurrence of lung cancer. However, she kept on smoking acknowledging that it was hazardous to her health. She often said to me "Ann, don't yell at me; I know that what I am doing is wrong". The instant she received news of another reoccurrence of the cancer, her long term partner made her leave his house, and she then became totally reliant on others to help her. Moreover, because of the reoccurrence of her cancer she became emotionally sober. Her mind became clearer; she finally accepted who loved her and the value of self.

Bernice was an Afro-American woman, who grew up in New York City. She was part of the generation who saw the segregation laws change and women's rights acknowledged. But she felt there was always an under current of segregation.

She spoke about how she went to an all-black school in New York City, had friends here and enjoyed it. Then, her mother sought something better for her and insisted upon her being bused to an all-white school in another part of the city. At that school, children would taunt her and make fun of her because she was one of the few black children that attended the school. The children there, perhaps unknowingly, showed her the threads of prejudice and bullying. Theses elements were woven into Bernice's unconscious cloth. Even as an adult, she still carried the feelings of hurt and shame.

Along with dealing with prejudice by others, she also had to cope with both physical and emotional abuse in her home. We often spoke about coping mechanisms and what she went through growing up, and even now confronting and dealing with similar situations as an adult woman. There were times the conversation would turns towards her relationship with men. She spoke of a pattern of falling in love over and over again with the "wrong type of man who did not want to commit to a relationship."

Her mother taught her different coping strategies to get through and survive in a world that was often hostile to her. Often, she found alcohol and smoking as a convenient way to cope with the difficulties that life presented. These habits added another thread to her cloth.

Every day was a challenge for her. Furthermore, there were many nagging questions that she always faced. Am I good enough for people to accept me? Who do I trust? Do I take care of my family or do I abandon them? Do I forgive those who have hurt me? How do I separate myself from toxic people in my life? How do I pay my healthcare bills that are so staggering?

At certain moments when she felt safe with me, she spoke abut her history and her thoughts about life.

Furthermore, even though she may have verbalized her concerns from time to time, her basic coping mechanism was "not to complain" and "just do what you have to do." Her emotional cloth was extremely fragile, and with each reoccurrence of cancer, she acknowledged the many physiological issues that affected her life.

However, emotional pain reaches deep into the psyche; intellectually, Bernice knew that she was a good person. Nonetheless, the small black child who faced adversity was still inside her, thinking, "if I keep quiet and do what I have to do, I will not get hurt." This childlike strategy for survival followed her despite her maturity as a grown woman. Bernice was still waiting to have permission from her to "grow up".

Joseph was an engaging, well-spoken, charming and attractive man. He took his cancer diagnosis calmly as part of his life's path. There was no anger or regrets about what he did or did not do. He was a wonderful family man and a great friend. His career was successful and it appeared that he was not facing any difficult financial circumstances.

As he would come in to receive his weekly chemotherapy, we usually would have discussions about politics, children or about life in general. One day, the conversation turned to stress and coping with it, and about how stress can increase the probability of getting cancer. I then said to him "But you don't have stress." He said, "What are you kidding me? I have a lot of stress. I had a mother who died from colon cancer at an early age. I have lived all my life with a sister who is schizophrenic. I am a caregiver for my sister and several elderly relatives in my family who depend on me. My wife had ovarian cancer; I am concerned that I will not be around to see my children settled in their lives. Plus, I have been undergoing chemotherapy for several years. Talk about stress". I saw in him the hidden thoughts and fears resulting from the emotional turmoil he was living though. Listening to him talk about his ancestry and how he was raised, I sensed a pattern of being stoic, of not letting people down. His mantra seemed to be keeping his fears hidden and not letting people know about them.

Our conversations also turned to spirituality as a way of coping with difficult situations. We both agreed that a person can be spiritual without being an observant follower of organized religion. When he was depressed or upset about his disease, I told him to go outside and feel the energy from the universe. To sit, and to see and feel the world around him. As he did this, he came to an understanding that all energies around us are also inside of us, and that peace and harmony do exist regardless of what you believe in. All you have to do is to be open-minded.

Katiya was born in The Soviet Union, into a family of diverse ethnic origins. Her mother's family never spoke about being Jewish until the Soviet Union fell and Russia became a separate republic.

During the breakup of the Soviet Union, her mother's cloth of having a Jewish background slowly started to reveal itself. Furthermore, because her mother was Jewish, this meant that Katiya was Jewish as well. Nevertheless, this information was guarded and not spoken of outside of the family for fear of prejudice or hostility by others.

Needless to say, Katiya lived a very austere life, while always watching her every word and movement out of fear of what might happen to her and of her family. At an early age, she was determined to be successful in all of her endeavors. She felt her life experiences made her stronger and that she could tolerate almost anything. Katiya was right; she was strong and very powerful. Her career enabled her to leave Russia, for global markets of the world. She was determined never to live a life of austerity again. Along the way, she fell in love and married.

The Jewish people have a proverb "People make plans and God laughs." Katiya had her life all figured out, past, present and future. However, there was a small caveat that was added to her life, one that she never foreseen. This was her "battle" with stomach cancer. Young, beautiful, active, and in her early thirties, she seemed to have a perfect life. Then she received her diagnosis of cancer. She attributed her cancer to having poor quality of food growing up in Russia. But was it all from poor quality of food? For several years she complained about stomach pain. She had tests done, without any indication of illness. However, she still maintained her demanding schedule, taking over the counter pills to help alleviate pain in her stomach. Not getting enough sleep added the thread of an unhealthy lifestyle to her emotional cloth. Her small intuitive voice slowly started to get louder and louder, making her aware that what she was doing was not working and urging her to pursue a different course of action.

Her perfect life had come to a screeching halt. All the answers that she thought she knew, no longer existed for her. She was placed in a domain that she never thought she would be in. More so, she began to look for a frame of reference to feel comfortable, to heal her emotional self. Her intuitive voice brought her to her ancestral Jewish thread of spirituality. She slowly discovered the concept of prayer for well being. From this exploration she felt calmness and solitude. More importantly, she achieved an inner tranquility that allowed her to move forward towards healing.

Over the many years I have worked in oncology, I have learned that money does not buy you happiness or contentment. Often I tell people to be careful what you wish for, all too often, people think money buys happiness. When you express your thoughts out loud about what you want and need, listen to the words and make sure that you have the whole perception of what you are looking for and what is important in your life. Interpretation and perception of what we think we need and want, and what the energies around us will bring to us, may be very different.

In the Unites States, there is no royalty; however, Irwin thought he was from a royal family. He came from a family that was prominent at one time and then because of various economic reasons, they lost their fortune. Irwin father's was a very demanding, controlling person, and at times abusive. He expected his son to do what he wanted him to do. However, as all children tend to do, Irwin sought out his own energies, which was likely disconcerting to his father.

He followed his intuitive instincts and became very successful in all of his endeavors. Wherever he went, he demanded and received respect because the power of his financial situation. His life was all about him, and controlling the players that he allowed into his court. Even with the best physicians and annual checkups, wholesome food and regular exercise, he was ultimately diagnosed with cancer.

Irwin was totally flabbergasted when he heard the words "You have cancer." This was not supposed to happen to him. The royal armor that Irwin built around himself was supposed to protect him from physical and emotional maladies. But cancer had reached even him and now he was reliant on others for his treatment and care.

Sometimes Irwin took off his royal armor and spoke to me about various topics. Far to often we tended to disagree on the subject matter. One particular day, he was extremely frustrated; he felt that people were talking about his care and making decisions without his impute. He was asking questions and no one was giving him answers. I acknowledged his frustration, and spoke with him about his situation. I explained that the first step in dealing with any illness is to recognize that you must be your own advocate. A patient should never be afraid to address specific questions to healthcare professionals and to people that are part of the healthcare team, regardless of the patient's stature. You always have control over your illness until you take your last breath. At that point he sat up in his chair and started to ask his physician specific questions regarding his care. Afterwards, I asked him if he felt better, and he said he did. His frustration was validated and he was able to speak on his own behalf regarding the progression of his care.

Connections, associations, links, ties relatives, acquaintances - - - there are so many words to describe an energy that shows how we are all influenced by each other. The essence of all this is to comprehend how all the threads are connected. A balanced of understanding of one's self, to validate what came before and to gain wisdom to help us move forward with physical and emotional health. Only when we gain this understanding can we attain, and find bliss in who we are.

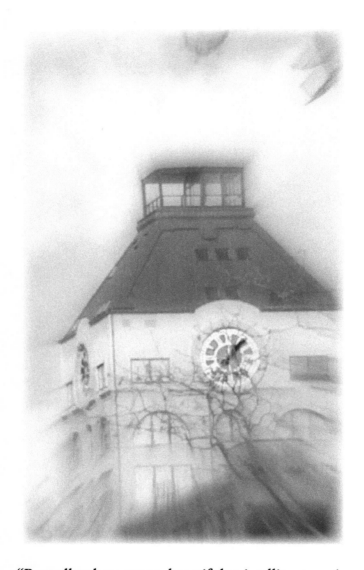

"Regardless how strong, beautiful or intelligent one is.
Time will come to decide how we will be remembered.
Respect others and create a legacy of love and kindness, for
in the end that is all we can give and take with us."

CHAPTER 13

YOU ARE NOT A FAILURE IF YOU DIE

Dr. Elizabeth Kubler-Ross was a world famous physician who researched the final stages of life and wrote many books on death and dying. She simplified the process that a person may go through as he or she faces death, classifying the process into "five stages of grief and dying."

The stages are:

- Denial: The initial stage: "it can't be happening."
- Anger: "Why Me?" It's not fair!" (either referring to God, oneself, or anybody perceived, rightly or wrongly, as "responsible")
- Bargaining: ("Just let me live to see my children graduate")
- Depression: "I'm so sad, why bother with anything?"
- Acceptance: "It's going to be OK."

Five Stages of Grief. Kübler-Ross, E. (1969) *On Death and Dying*, Routledge, ISBN 0-415-04015-9

I believe that there is another stage that we go through when we start to accept the process of dying. It is characterized by a sense of disappointment, by a feeling of having fallen short of what was expected of you, anxiety and trepidations about dying.

Here are some of the thoughts and feelings that you may experience

- Am I a failure because I did not conquer this disease?
- Am I giving up by accepting the fact that I am going to die?
- Am I a failure because I let people down?
- Am I a failure because I will not be there for my family and friends in the future?
- Am I a financial burden because of the costly bills, tests and expense that were spent on me?
- My dreams and aspirations won't be fulfilled.
- Failure of not maintaining a good relationship, with friends and family.
- The fear of not being remembered
- The fear of the unknown
- The fear of pain
- Regrets
- I am not a good role model for my children, friends and family if I give up this "fight"?
- Will this be the right decision for more religiously?

There are no right or wrong answers on how to cope with these feelings. But there must be an understanding within you that the survival for life must stop. By letting go of the quest to sustain life and by allowing the natural process of dying to come into your life, you still have the capability to make your life fulfilling and worthy even at the final stages of end of life.

When we face our own mortality and realize that our death may happen today, we suddenly become poets, lovers, philosophers and diplomats. We discover what really is important to us and what matters most.

When a person enters the end of life stage, they must go through the stages of death and dying. Furthermore, so must friends and family when they hear this type of news. It is essential that all who are involved in your life, must go through the emotionally stages of death and dying as well. One must be aware of friends and family may not communicate how upset they are and may hide these feelings from the person that is passing.

It is a person's prerogative to keep seeking the formula for wellness and good health. But comprehend the mindset of all loved ones who will do anything for the one who is passing to keep the person here with them. The transition will be less difficult for everyone, by allowing people to voice their sadness and grief.

Before the transition of the end stages of life, there should be a discussion and clearly make it known to everyone who will be affected, the wishes of the person who will be passing. Simply, there should be no surprises or arguments or regrets from others, it your wishes are known.

For those who are in the process of dealing with the stages of end of life, you have a choice to allow yourself to let go life's energy. By doing so, you unintentionally take on a role as a teacher showing the acceptance of death with dignity. You are teaching people around you about dying and the lessons of the importance of love and compassion. The greatest eternal gift is love, this is what you can give and receive. It will always be cherished because your students will always have your gift within them, and will be able to feel your presence at all times.

My mother made the decision to be placed in a hospital setting for her final days of her life. It was an excellent and caring place designed for cancer patients. At the end of her days, she did not want to see anyone other than her immediate family and felt that this was a safe haven for her. My mother never had any physical pain from cancer. Her pain was emotional.

Because of the advanced stage of her disease, and the fact that she was in a hospital, she was able to get intravenous hydration. As a nurse, she was very well aware that her bodily functions were starting to shut down and she needed this hydration to survive. Out of anger, depression, and frustration she asked for someone to take her life. For her, this was no way to live.

Every day, when I went to visit with her, she expressed her thoughts of having someone take her life; she would get angry with me when I reminded her that no one wanted to do that for or to her. Then on one of my visits, I pointed out to her that she should speak with her healthcare team and stop the daily intravenous hydrations. I emphasized to her that she still had the capability and the power to make her own decisions about her life.

The next time I saw her, she told me that she had spoken with her healthcare team and she was stopping the hydration. After she made that decision, I watched a rapid decline in my mother's health. She was still able to talk, but she was getting weaker and weaker. I knew that my mother was in the final stage of her life.

The last time I saw my mother, it was during one of my routine daily visits with her. However, that particular day I felt this strange energy around my mother's bed and around me. She was slipping in and out of consciousness. She was reaching out with her hands as if she was taking to someone, but there was no one there other than myself in the room. It was time for me to go, I said good-bye to her and told her that I loved her, and I would see her the next day. But somehow, when I left her, I knew in my heart that I was never going to see her again. I received a telephone call from her doctor that my mother passed away peacefully later that evening.

My sister Lois dealt with the challenges of cancer for five years. How she maintained her optimistic point of view about life, despite surgery, grueling chemotherapy, countless tests, and many abdominal taps was amazing. Somehow, she always found the strength to dance, travel, and spend time with her family and friends. She made every day a special day for her.

During those years, she experienced a steady decline of quality of life. But to see Lois, she looked like the "picture of health" often her own family was fooled by her appearance of beauty, strength and athletic ability. We all thought Lois was like the "Energizer Battery Bunny," she kept going despite the obstacles that were facing her.

Denial was a great coping mechanism for me, even though deep in my heart, I knew the impending outcome for Lois. Especially, when I saw her eighty-pound body and I realized that her passing was inevitable.

As she was approaching her final hours, she expressed many feelings to me. She asked the proverbial question of "Why me?" with anger. Another feeling she had was of failure, because she did not conquer her disease. Furthermore, she was overwhelmed with guilt for being a burden on her family. Another feeling was that she was being punished because she hurt someone, and it was bad Karma coming back to her. Even though I reassured her that what she felt was untrue, she still had misgivings.

I stayed by her side, which she found very comforting. We were sisters and we both needed each other. I needed to be there for her, and she needed me to help to alleviate the fear of the unknown. However, her husband was still in denial of what was going to happen to Lois. He was her "hero", and he was going to revive her health. For him, he thought food would make her feel better. What he did not comprehend was that when a person is dying, giving food to them does not make them feel better. In her heart she did not have the strength to tell him to stop and to accept what was happening to her. She asked me to tell him not to feed her anymore or prepare food for her. However, I told her that she must be the one to do so. She still had the strength of mind to be her own advocate and to make her own decisions for herself. Therefore, by addressing the issue, it showed her that she still had the ability to be in control of her own life that was unraveling hour by hour. More importantly, by speaking to him, it helped him to recognize what was happening to her.

She gathered up her courage and spoke with him alone. The food issue ceased and he understood what she wanted in her final hours. During her last twenty-four hours of life, she became pensive, and we began to reminisce about our childhood, our weddings, our parents, our siblings' and our children. By this time, she only felt remorse that she would not be part of her daughters' lives. Moreover, she expressed gratitude that she had a "wonderful life."

Lois took her last breathe with her family at her bedside. I said good-bye to my sister as well and saw that she was at peace.

During the final stages of prostate cancer, my father-in-law did not have the strength to get out of bed. However, he still prayed daily, told jokes and conversed with friends and family.

Somehow, he must have been cognizant that his time for passing was near. Hence, one day he and I were alone together. He started to talk to me about the upcoming four Jewish holidays that were going to take place in the next few weeks. He went through each holiday until he got to the last one. He then looked at me and said, "It will be the end."

On the eve of the fourth and final Jewish holiday of Simchat Torah, my father-in-law began to slip away. I told him that it was the beginning of the holiday and he nodded to me. As his family saw that his end was near, they gathered around his bedside, each telling him how much they loved him and how they would miss him. On this particular holiday, the Jewish people gathered in synagogue's to celebrate the love and the privilege of completing the cycle of reading the entire Torah over the course of a year and starting anew, once again, with the reading of GENESIS.

My father-in-law's profound spiritual message about continuation of love and the meaning of life was his way to bring comfort to his children and to his grandchildren. Throughout the holiday, I was with him. Periodically, I spoke with him and he nodded acknowledging that he understood what I was saying to him. Finally early Sunday morning, the last day of the holiday I explained to him that it was the last day. I took his hand, he nodded, and then I told him that it was okay to let go and to pass on.

After nearly 48 hours at his side, my husband and I left to go home for a brief rest, expecting to return later. As we arrived home, we received the telephone call that he passed away.

I hope that sharing these private moments about my family members and their passing, will help the reader to have a better comprehension that you always have choices in life. Even though they may be difficult ones to make.

The end of life decisions should be spoken about way before anyone gets in a situation, where they are unable to speak their wishes. This book is primary about cancer patients and the emphasis that they must communicate their wishes of how they want to live and during the end stages of life regarding how they want to pass.

Over the years I have council many families to allow their loved ones to pass on with dignity. Needless to say there have been times when the emotions of a family member or friend over powers what I call a "good death". They will insist to have extraordinary measures to maintain life support for them regardless of what they expressed for end of life decisions.

It may appear to be a selfish act that the family member or friend has by not letting go of the love one. Or, perhaps if may be do to fear, or loneliness or anxiety if there loved one is really at "peace". Trying to find answers some people seek out psychics, soothsayers or have vivid dreams about their loved one. Trying to find the answers are very difficult for the grieving person.

These thoughts and actions will prevail. Often people will say to them "get over it" or "time heals all wounds" or "move forward and slowly you will forget." Those comforting words for me are not comforting. When you lose a love one to any circumstances it is very hard to move forward.

What I tell friends and family members, you don't have to forget. Acknowledged your grief, but don't allow your grief from stopping you from living a full and contented life. I truly can say, that I know that your loved ones would not want you to be depressed about them passing. On the contrary, what they wanted for you in your life still holds true.

For you to be loved, and to receive love back. Enjoy every moment of every day. In addition to that, walk as if their spirit is next to you. No one can truly say that they are not with you.

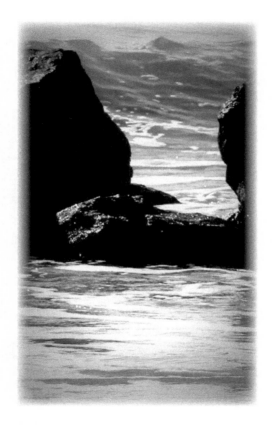

"Looking back with regrets and remorse is not the code for healing. Take a lesson from the universe. It has the extraordinary ability of forever changing and moving forward with grace. So must you."

CHAPTER 14

RENEWAL CONTRACT FOR WELL-BEING

Consciously and unconsciously you are sending out messages to your family, friends and to your healthcare team about what you expect and need from them to help you. Furthermore you are also sending a subtext of messages connecting how you've managed to live with cancer. These internal subtest messages have been shown to make a difference in your over all outlook in life.

To help overcome the negative internal subtext or scripts/negative baggage, you must renew your own inner well being. Regardless of what your prognosis may be, you still can change your internal thoughts and gain a feeling of calmness and a sense of well being.

There are many ways to accomplish this. However, the easiest way is to write down words that are relevant to you. Take the word "CANCER" and replace it with another "C" word or words that make you feel good. Try doing this every day when you wake up. Think of this as Renewal Contract for your inner well being. The best part about this contract is that it can be done every day, without anyone knowing but you.

Another part of this Renewal Contract for your inner well being is to comprehend to take one day at a time. There are many things that we cannot control in our lives. Nevertheless, we are each capable of controlling our minds, our feelings and the knowledge that everyone lives just one day at a time.

Here are words that being with the letter **C** that can be used to replace the word **"cancer:"**

Courage	**Community**	**Conscious**
Cheer	**Compassion**	**Cooperation**
Charity	**Chemotherapy**	**Creative**
Cure	**Complete**	**Transformation**
Cerebral	**Cognizance**	**Confusion**
Comedy	**Cantaloupes**	**Cup**
Communicate	**Competence**	**Caring**
Chocolate	**Creativity**	**Coach**
Connection	**Conveyance**	**Code**
Chopin	**Challenge**	**Celebration**
Clarity	**Conduct**	**Cucumbers**
Contribution	**Clever**	**Closeness**
Consistency	**Cope**	**Chaplin**
Cuddle	**Chrysalis**	**Cosmos**
Chaotic	**Caretaker**	**Cloud**
Causes	**Control**	

A mother bought her daughter a box of animal crackers that she begged for while grocery shopping. She spread out the animal shaped crackers all over the kitchen table. "What are you doing?" her Mother asked. "The box says you can't eat them if the seal is broken." The little girl explained, "I am looking for the seal."

We all experience trying to follow directions and looking for the seal to make things work for us. But there is our intuitive voice inside all of us that does give us directions. We just have to be more aware of what it is saying to us. Ignoring it and keeping it a small voice does not work. For in the end it does get louder as we move along into maladies that we don't want.

One of my sayings that I have learned from life's lessons for me is, "Pay attention to life's small lessons and learn from them. For if you don't you will get bigger ones and harder ones to learn from."

As an oncology nurse for many years and someone who has helped patients get through life changing experiences, I believe patients develop a "subconscious film" in their minds to help them cope with their disease. From my own observations, there are usually three scenes and subplots (added when necessary) that pertain to specific defense mechanism to help the transition. Furthermore, patients take on such interchangeable roles, as director or editor, in order to change the various scenes in their "subconscious film" to gain greater control of their life and their disease process. Just as in making a real film, the ability to keep filming pause, edit, re-write and add special effects are necessary elements to help our inner psyche get though difficult moments in our lives. At certain times, it might be advantageous to keep filming, and at other times it may be necessary to stop, due to many different reasons such as anxiety, sadness or stress. I feel that by, making a "subconscious film" a person somehow has the ability to develop and to maintain good coping skills that are necessary to reach a healthy emotional outcome.

The concept that cancer is a disease always resulting in death is changing in our society. Furthermore, due to better diagnostic tests and advanced chemotherapy modalities, cancer has become a chronic disease for many people. Bobbi was diagnosed with three different primary tumors in her life. Each time she visited her physicians, she was subjected to various treatments for her cancer. Because of her experiences with cancer, she now has "flashbacks" of what she went through while she was undergoing different cancer modalities. Usually, these memories occur when she is getting closer to the time of her annual visits to her physicians.

A "subconscious film" starts in her mind about her life before, during and after cancer. She is afraid of her examination because of "what if"... What if the doctor finds another cancer in her body? To help her deal with her different cancer she had read and taken many classes regarding coping strategies for her well being.

Over that period of time, she has learned that "flashbacks" do happen (it is a normal process and now she knows to take one day at a time. In addition to that, when she feels the anxiety inside her body, she uses several coping strategies to help her. One techniques is changing the word "cancer" into "C" words that are funny sounding and pleasant to her.

Another coping technique that she uses before her examination is making up a list in her mind all the things that she is grateful for. This reduces her anxiety and gives her inner strength and a feeling of well being when she faces her doctor.

When she gets her "clean bill" of health from her doctor, she calls all her children to tell them the good news. Then she breaths a sigh of appreciation for living another year and being able to enjoy and see her friends and family. Before her cancer, she was appreciative of her life and of her surroundings. However, because of her cancers she now feels more alive than she was before she had this disease.

Sometimes, kismet does come into play regarding your sense of well being and you do get a second chance to find happiness. This happened to Sylvia, who was a wonderful wife and mother for over forty years. During the last five years of her marriage, she became her husband's caretaker while he underwent surgery and chemotherapy. However, it was unfortunate that he did not live to experience the newer treatments for colon cancer and he died. This difficult experience had a profound effect on Sylvia, which I noticed when I met her. She was very anxious about undergoing her own chemotherapy for colon cancer. Every time I would see her in the office, she always had tears in her eyes, because of the flashback of her husband's experience. Along with that, she felt as if she was at the bottom of a "very deep black hole" and she felt that she was unable to climb out from it.

During the months while Sylvia was undergoing chemotherapy, she would speak about her loving husband and their relationship together, apparently, they built a successful small business and had the ability to help people in need. She was angry at God for allowing "such a good person" like her husband to go through the ordeal of cancer therapy and not be cured. Furthermore, she felt that she was being punished because she lost her loving husband, and now she, too, had coon cancer.

Over time, she saw that she had an easier time with her chemotherapy than her husband did. This gave her a different perspective on what her outcome would be. Gradually, she started to feel that she was not at the bottom of her "black hole" there were some rays of sunshine coming though. However, she still was angry at God for taking away such a good person as her husband.

One evening she went out to dinner with her girlfriends at a local restaurant; they were laughing and having a good time. One of her girlfriends mentioned her name out loud and an elderly man came over to the table to see if he knew Sylvia. It turned out that he knew Sylvia when she was a young girl living in Bronx, New York. He always wondered what happened to her and could not believe hearing her name that evening. After all those years, they were both delighted to see each other and started to reminisce.

That particular dinner became a very special one for Sylvia. Her old friend Herbie became a very important person in her life. Over the course of time, she discovered that he lost his wife to cancer, and he was wondering whatever happened to her. He thought it was very fortuitous for him to find her in that restaurant that particular night.

More rays of sunshine came through to Sylvia. During the course of her chemotherapy treatments she and Herbie fell in love and made plans to be married.

Sylvia and Herbie had a beautiful wedding together after her chemotherapy. They went on a romantic honeymoon to Paris. Her feeling of desperation and despair that once felt before and during her chemotherapy had changed. Her "black hole" became a surreal memory of her, and now, she found happiness. Her anger towards God changed into being thankful for having Herbie in her life.

A great deal of time is consumed by cancer patients while undergoing different types of cancer modalities and focusing on a good outcome. Therefore familiarities and comfort level is formed by some patients because of this routine. Difficulty may occur for theses patients when they have to move on to another phase in their life after their cancer modalities are over. Often they may feel a "post-treatment letdown" or ask, "What do I do next?"

Because of this letdown, for many patients the completion of chemotherapy is bittersweet. They are relieved that the ordeal is over and happy to be finished with their treatments, but they have formed a special bond with the staff and the physicians and will miss them. Often I ask patients "What are you going to do to change your life?" Or "How are you going to maintain your inner well being?" Many of the patients are surprised when I ask them theses questions because they never questioned themselves about life after treatments. By putting these questions to them, they start to reflect on life before during and after cancer.

When I meet someone, I say, "Pay attentions to life's lessons and learn from them. For if you don't you will get bigger ones to learn from." There are many patients that I have taken care of over the years that I feel this saying applies too. But there is one particular patient that sums up all of the stories that are in this book and my quote about life.

Marisa was a small, quiet woman whose mother was an immigrant and father was an American citizen and lived in New York City. During her childhood years, she was expected to do well in school, help in the home, be quiet when her father comes home from work and be courteous to others. One day, along came her "Prince Charming" and the answer to getting out of her parents" house. She married her "Prince Charming and the first years of her marriage went well. Her husband was still her "Prince Charming" until children came along. His demeanor began to change and he became more demanding, which later turned into verbal abuse.

She stayed with her husband even though she was unhappy with her situation because she felt it was the right thing to do. Living with him was extremely difficult for her, but she was not physically abusive towards her so she felt secure that she would be okay and no harm would come to her. However, she was always on "pins and needles" because of the tension associated with living with her husband.

She got a job, which she enjoyed very much, and it became her safe haven from her husband. Her co-workers respected her, which was difficult for her to comprehend. However, she still went home to a controlling, abusive husband, and never showed her animosity towards him. Over the years, she became robotic and just went through the motions of being a good wife and mother, trying to keep "peace" in the household for her children. Food became her comfort to help ease the tension.

Living in a stressful relationship with her husband started to take a physical toll on her body. She gained weight and suffered from an unhealthy physical and emotional lifestyle. She still was stoic and refused to change. However, she still did not want to challenge her husband regarding his abusive behavior, because she still wanted to maintain peace in the house, She tried to get into a routine of diet and exercise, but found that it was difficult to do. He life became so overwhelming and she had a heart attack because of stress and her obesity.

Marisa's heart attack was a bigger "wake-up call" than her weight issues. Hence she realized the need to start changing her life to get well. Knowing that her relationship with her husband was unhealthy for her, she made several attempts to get him to change his behavior. However, fear of getting another heart attack she ultimately gave up and did not confront him any further about his attitude. Once again it was important to maintain peace in the home.

Her third "wake-up call" came one morning when she felt a lump underneath her arm. The lump turned out be a cancerous lymph node and now she was looking at an even bigger challenge regarding her life. She told her husband about the outcome of her examination, thinking that he would finally stop his destructive behavior towards her. Instead, he essentially told her that he did not care about her and left the room.

On the first day of chemotherapy treatment, she was very anxious because she did know what to expect. She could not believe that this surreal dream was reality. Moreover, because of her cancer she was now confronting her own mortality, whereas with other health issues, she never gave it much thought. Furthermore, she felt remorse that her husband was not with her to support her through such a difficult time.

As Marisa was undergoing her chemotherapy sessions, her world slowly started to change. Now, she began to see a new image of herself. She saw herself as a bud, which slowly opened into a flower. As each petal unfurled she envisioned friends, family members, co-workers and her healthcare team as part of her flower. All the petals surrounded her; she was in the center of a flower of healing and well being. Slowly, she started to comprehend the important concept of "I, myself" and to heal her inner being.

Throughout her life, she was quiet and never looked for fanfare or gratitude from other people when she would help them. Now, because of her cancer, there has been an outpouring from people due to her kindness towards them when the needed help. She acknowledged to me that was supposed to be a very dark moment in her life actually turned out to be one of the brightest moment in it. Unintentionally, she is facing her mortality with strength, courage and pride in who she is. Somehow, through her cancer, she found inner peace and a safe haven within herself.

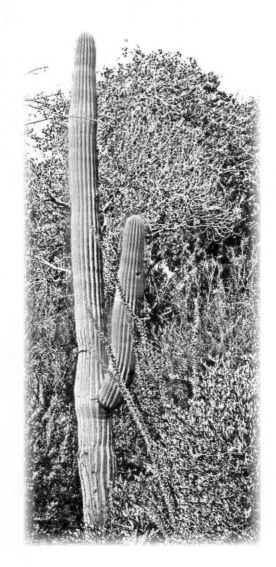

"In nature the Saguaro cactus has the ability to heal itself from within. You have this extraordinary power to do the same, use it."

Postscript

Looking?

When cancer or serious illness affects us via ourselves, our family members or friends, we inadvertently start the process of seeking some form of comfort to help alleviate the difficult times we anticipate that we are going to have or just having. Over the years I have seen people seek out all types of physical and spiritual modalities, believing that these modalities will help with their "cure".

Perhaps they do work. It is not up to me to second guess anyone on what is best for them on how they are dealing with their illness. However, the analogy that I use with my patients to understand that they have the ability to "heal themselves" is the story of Dorothy in the Wizard of Oz.

As you read the story, Dorothy has many experiences trying to find her way back home. Along her journey she encounters, many different types of experiences. At times it was fun, other times very dangerous. However, as she pursue ways to get back home-asking help from other people; it became clearer to her that they did not have the power to help her get back home.

Just at the moment when Dorothy lost hope of ever returning to her "way of life" the "good witch" appeared. The "good witch" explained to Dorothy, she had the power to return home (the safe place) the whole time she was in a strange land.

All of us have the capacity to find home, a safe place. Our home is inside all of us. It is a place that will give us courage, kindness, and the mental capacity to help heal ourselves from within. All we have to do is just close our eye and click our heels, three times and find our home.

It is that simple.

REFLECTIVE THOUGHTS

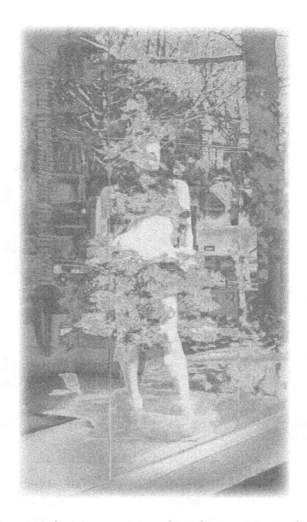

"Emotional scars are our goods and trimmings to dress the window of our unconsciousness. The choice to incorporate them and to allow them to enhance our life experiences is up to the dresser of our consciousness."

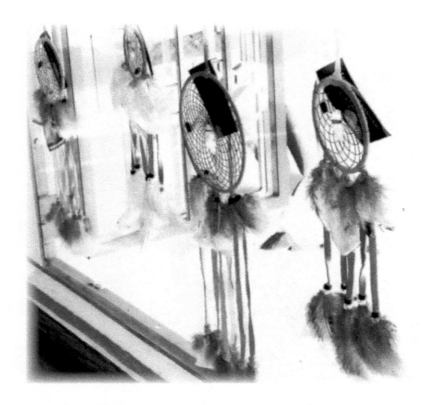

"Nightmares are dreams. These difficult dreams give you
the thought process to acknowledge what frightens you.
Catch them, understand them and discard them."

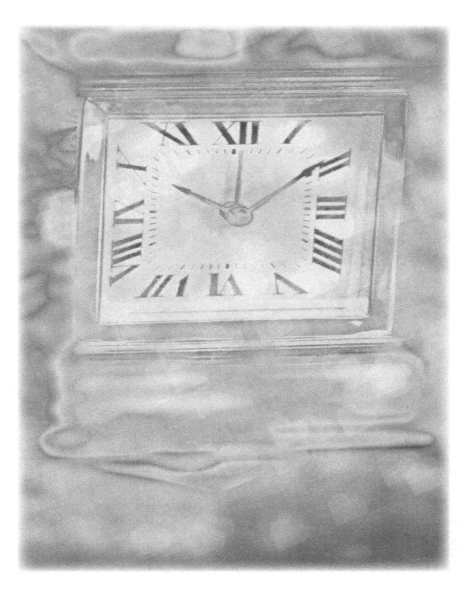

"The perception that time heals all wounds is just
an illusion. We just learn how to hide the wounds
more effectively and move forward in life."

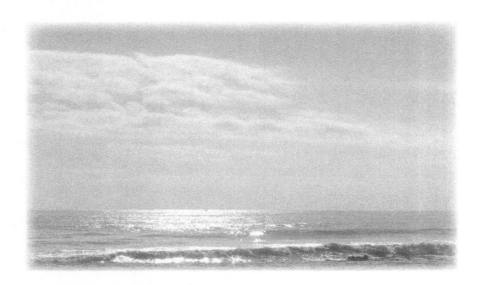

"The tides of the ocean have an ever-changing script. But the ability to maintain its beauty and spirituality is there regardless."

ABOUT THE AUTHOR

Ann Wax has been a healthcare professional for over 35 years, as Registered Nurse, a health educator and a consultant; her specialties include oncology nursing, health education, stress relief and positive mindfulness. She has been quoted in the Huffington Post on "Tips for Cancer" as well as speaking at Gilda's Clubs, Barnes and Noble, colleges and many community organizations. Her new book "Op-Ed on Cancer" brings together helpful advice from her point of view and from her patients' on coping strategies to get through the surreal dream of cancer.